# Education and the General Surgeon

*Editor*

PAUL J. SCHENARTS

# SURGICAL CLINICS
# OF NORTH AMERICA

www.surgical.theclinics.com

*Consulting Editor*
RONALD F. MARTIN

August 2021 • Volume 101 • Number 4

ELSEVIER

1600 John F. Kennedy Boulevard • Suite 1800 • Philadelphia, Pennsylvania, 19103-2899

http://www.surgical.theclinics.com

**SURGICAL CLINICS OF NORTH AMERICA Volume 101, Number 4**
**August 2021 ISSN 0039–6109, ISBN-13: 978-0-323-81374-7**

Editor: John Vassallo, j.vassallo@elsevier.com
Developmental Editor: Arlene Campos

*Surgical Clinics of North America* (ISSN 0039–6109) is published bimonthly by Elsevier Inc., 360 Park Avenue South, New York, NY 10010-1710. Months of publication are February, April, June, August, October, and December. Business and Editorial Offices: 1600 John F. Kennedy Blvd., Suite 1800, Philadelphia, PA 19103-2899. Periodicals postage paid at New York, NY and additional mailing offices. Subscription prices are $443.00 per year for US individuals, $1198.00 per year for US institutions, $100.00 per year for US & Canadian students and residents, $547.00 per year for Canadian individuals, $1270.00 per year for Canadian institutions, $536.00 for international individuals, $1270.00 per year for international institutions and $250.00 per year for foreign students/residents. To receive student/resident rate, orders must be accompanied by name of affiliated institution, date of term, and the *signature* of program/residency coordinator on institution letterhead. Orders will be billed at individual rate until proof of status is received. Foreign air speed delivery is included in all *Clinics* subscription prices. All prices are subject to change without notice. POSTMASTER: Send address changes to *Surgical Clinics*, Elsevier Health Sciences Division, Subscription Customer Service, 3251 Riverport Lane, Maryland Heights, MO 63043. **Customer Service (orders, claims, online, change of address): Telephone: 1-800-654-2452 (U.S. and Canada); 314-447-8871 (outside U.S. and Canada). Fax: 314-447-8029. E-mail: journalscustomerservice-usa@elsevier.com (for print support); journalsonlinesupport-usa@elsevier.com (for online support).**

*Reprints.* For copies of 100 or more, of articles in this publication, please contact the Commercial Reprints Department, Elsevier Inc., 360 Park Avenue South, New York, New York 10010-1710. Tel. 212-633-3874, Fax: 212-633-3820, E-mail: reprints@elsevier.com.

*The Surgical Clinics of North America* is also published in Spanish by McGraw-Hill Interamericana Editores S.A., P.O. Box 5-237 06500 Mexico D.F. Mexico; and in Portuguese by Interlivros Edicoes Ltda., Rua Comandante Coelho 1085, CEP 21250, Rio de Janeiro, Brazil; and in Greek by Paschalidis Medical Publications, Athens Greece.

*The Surgical Clinics of North America* is covered in *MEDLINE/PubMed (Index Medicus)*, *EMBASE/Excerpta Medica*, *Current Contents/Clinical Medicine*, *Current Contents/Life Sciences*, *Science Citation Index*, and *ISI/BIOMED*.

# Contributors

## CONSULTING EDITOR

**RONALD F. MARTIN, MD, FACS**
Colonel (Retired), United States Army Reserve; General and HPB Surgeon, Department of General Surgery and Surgical Oncology, Madigan Army Medical Center, Tacoma, Washington

## EDITOR

**PAUL J. SCHENARTS, MD, FACS**
Professor and Associate Dean for Clinical Affairs, Des Moines University, College of Osteopathic Medicine, Des Moines, Iowa; Professor of Surgery, Creighton University, School of Medicine, Omaha, Nebraska

## AUTHORS

**JENNIFER S. BEATY, MD, FACS, FASCRS**
Associate Dean of Student Advancement and Graduate Medical Education, Assistant Professor of Surgery, Des Moines University College of Osteopathic Medicine, Des Moines, Iowa

**DAVID L. BOUWMAN, MD, FACS**
Professor Emeritus, The Michael and Marian Ilitch Department of Surgery, Wayne State University School of Medicine, Detroit, Michigan

**DANIEL L. DENT, MD, FACS**
Professor, UT Health San Antonio, Department of Surgery, San Antonio, Texas

**SEAN DIEFFENBAUGHER, MD**
Assistant Professor, Carolinas Medical Center, Atrium Health, Department of Surgery, Charlotte, North Carolina

**DAVID A. EDELMAN, MD, MSHPEd, FACS**
Professor of Surgery, The Michael and Marian Ilitch Department of Surgery, Wayne State University School of Medicine, Detroit, Michigan

**FUMIKO EGAWA, MD, FACS, FASCRS**
Department of Surgery, Creighton University School of Medicine, Omaha, Nebraska

**JUDITH FRENCH, PhD**
Surgical Education Researcher, Cleveland Clinic, Cleveland, Ohio

**JEFFREY M. GAUVIN, MD, MS, FACS**
Department of Surgical Education, Santa Barbara, California

**AMY HAN, MD**
Surgical Education Research Fellow, Cleveland Clinic, Cleveland, Ohio

**QUINTON MORROW HATCH, MD**
Madigan Army Medical Center, General Surgery, Tacoma, Washington

**ADITI JALLA, MD**
University of Oklahoma Health Sciences Center College of Medicine, Department of Surgery, Oklahoma City, Oklahoma

**MUNEERA R. KAPADIA, MD, MME**
Department of Surgery, The University of North Carolina at Chapel Hill, Chapel Hill, North Carolina

**JASON W. KEMPENICH, MD, FACS**
Associate Professor, UT Health San Antonio, Department of Surgery, San Antonio, Texas

**TATYANA KOPILOVA, MD**
Department of Surgical Education, Santa Barbara, California

**IAN KRATZKE, MD**
Department of Surgery, The University of North Carolina at Chapel Hill, Chapel Hill, North Carolina

**JASON LEES, MD**
University of Oklahoma Health Sciences Center College of Medicine, Department of Surgery, Oklahoma City, Oklahoma

**JEREMY LIPMAN, MD, MHPE**
Program Director of General Surgery Residency, Cleveland Clinic, Cleveland, Ohio

**CALLIE D. McADAMS, MD**
Division of Vascular Surgery, Department of Surgery, University of Tennessee, Knoxville, Tennessee

**MICHAEL M. McNALLY, MD, FACS**
Division of Vascular Surgery, Associate Professor, Department of Surgery, University of Tennessee, Knoxville, Tennessee

**LILAH F. MORRIS-WISEMAN, MD, FACS**
Associate Professor, Surgery, Associate Program Director, General Surgery Residency, Department of Surgery, University of Arizona, Tucson, Arizona

**VALENTINE N. NFONSAM, MD, MS, FACS, FASCRS**
Professor of Surgery, Program Director, General Surgery Residency, Interim Chief, Division of Surgical Oncology, Department of Surgery, University of Arizona, Tucson, Arizona

**LEAH PLUMBLEE, MD**
Medical University of South Carolina, Department of Surgery, Charleston, South Carolina

**JACOB A. QUICK, MD, FACS**
Department of Surgery, Division of Acute Care Surgery, University of Missouri, Columbia, Missouri

**KARI M. ROSENKRANZ, MD**
Associate Professor, Department of Surgery, Dartmouth Geisel School of Medicine, Dartmouth-Hitchcock Medical Center, Lebanon, New Hampshire

**PAUL J. SCHENARTS, MD, FACS**
Professor and Associate Dean for Clinical Affairs, Des Moines University, College of Osteopathic Medicine, Des Moines, Iowa; Professor of Surgery, Creighton University, School of Medicine, Omaha, Nebraska

**RACHEL E. SCHENKEL, MD**
Department of Surgery, Creighton University, School of Medicine, Omaha, Nebraska

**RICHARD A. SIDWELL, MD, FACS**
Former Program Director of General Surgery Residency, Iowa Methodist Medical Center, Des Moines, Iowa; Adjunct Clinical Professor, Department of Surgery, University of Iowa Carver College of Medicine, Iowa City, Iowa

**VANCE YOUNG SOHN, MD**
Department of Surgery, Madigan Army Medical Center, Joint Base Lewis McChord, Washington

**CAMERON ST. HILAIRE, MD**
Department of Surgical Education, Santa Barbara, California

**RYLAND STUCKE, MD**
Fellow in Advanced GI and Minimally Invasive Surgery, Department of Surgery, Oregon Health and Science University, Portland, Oregon

**JOURDAN STURGES, BS**
University of Oklahoma Health Sciences Center College of Medicine, Department of Surgery, Oklahoma City, Oklahoma

**MAURA E. SULLIVAN, PhD**
Department of Surgery, University of Southern California, Los Angeles, California

**CYNTHIA TALLEY, MD, FACS**
Vice Chair of Education, Associate Professor, Medical University of South Carolina, Department of Surgery, Charleston, South Carolina

**SAMANTHA L. TARRAS, MD, FACS**
Assistant Professor of Surgery, The Michael and Marian Ilitch Department of Surgery, Wayne State University School of Medicine, Detroit, Michigan

**JOCK THACKER, MD**
Surgery Resident, The Michael and Marian Ilitch Department of Surgery, Wayne State University School of Medicine, Detroit, Michigan

**CHRISTOPHER THOMAS, MD**
Medical University of South Carolina, Department of Surgery, Charleston, South Carolina

**LAUREL A. VAUGHAN, MD**
Department of Surgery, Division of Acute Care Surgery, University of Missouri, Columbia, Missouri

**MICHAEL MINH VU, MD**
Madigan Army Medical Center, General Surgery, Tacoma, Washington

**JESSICA BRITTANY WEISS, MD**
Madigan Army Medical Center, General Surgery, Tacoma, Washington

# Contents

**Foreword: Surgical Education**     xiii

Ronald F. Martin

**Preface: Surgical Education**     xvii

Paul J. Schenarts

**The Biology and Psychology of Surgical Learning**     541

Paul J. Schenarts, Rachel E. Schenkel, and Maura E. Sullivan

Surgical education requires proficiency with multiple types of learning to create capable surgeons. This article reviews a conceptual framework of learning that starts with the biological basis of learning and how neural networks encode memory. We then focus on how information can be absorbed, organized, and recalled, discussing concepts such as cognitive load, knowledge retrieval, and adult learning. Influences on memory and learning such as stress, sleep, and unconscious bias are explored. This overview of the biological and psychological aspects to learning provides a foundation for the articles to follow.

**Teaching on Rounds and in Small Groups**     555

Christopher Thomas, Leah Plumblee, Sean Dieffenbaugher, and Cynthia Talley

Bedside teaching plays a vital role in training future physicians, allowing for instruction in history taking, physical examination skills, differential diagnosis development, professionalism, teamwork integration, effective communication, and discussions of medical ethics. Due to changes in the health care system, accreditation bodies, and shortened admittance of patients, rates of bedside teaching have declined. Attending surgeons feel increased external pressures to meet performance metrics while resident physicians adhere to duty hour restrictions. This article highlights popular methods, including bedside rounds, near-peer teaching, and resident versus attending preceptors, and discusses how teaching on rounds has an impact on patients.

**Effective Large Group Teaching for General Surgery**     565

Samantha L. Tarras, Jock Thacker, David L. Bouwman, and David A. Edelman

Large group settings display no signs of disappearing. Most surgeons charged with this education have received no formal training. Lecturing remains the most common method of educating large groups. Even though factors required for an excellent lecture are known, their inconsistent application results in variation of effectiveness. Long-standing principles of rhetoric and recent advances in neuroscience, cognitive science, learning models, and teaching theory play a role in achieving effectiveness. This article makes recommendations for creating and delivering lectures, including active learning opportunities and modern innovations in information technology supporting teaching methods. Effective lecturing skills are acquired by persistent deliberate practice.

**Teaching and Evaluating Nontechnical Skills for General Surgery**        577

Ryland Stucke and Kari M. Rosenkranz

Surgical training programs have long used quantitative measures of knowledge, as well as subjective evaluation of technical skills, to define the competence of trainees. However, a growing body of literature has shown the importance of nontechnical surgical skills as vital components of quality surgical care. Institutions must train nontechnical surgical skills, including leadership, communication, teamwork, situational awareness, and decision making, and incorporate these attributes into their evaluative processes to maximally enhance surgical performance at every career stage.

**Intraoperative Teaching and Evaluation in General Surgery**        587

Richard A. Sidwell

The operating room continues to be the location where surgical residents develop both technical and nontechnical skills, ultimately culminating with them being capable of safe and independent practice. The process of intraoperative instruction is, by necessity, moving from an apprentice-based model where skills are acquired somewhat randomly through repeated exposure and evaluation is done in a global gestalt fashion. Modern surgical education demands that intraoperative instruction be intentional and that evaluation provides formative and summative feedback. This chapter describes some best practice approaches to intraoperative teaching and evaluation.

**General Surgery Resident Autonomy: Truth and Myth**        597

Jason W. Kempenich and Daniel L. Dent

Within general surgery education circles, the state of autonomy for residents in surgery training programs has been of growing concern. Although there is no direct evidence showing less autonomy in modern surgical training, multiple surrogates have been cited as reasons for concern. Many reasons have been given for lost autonomy including the 80-hour work week, financial constraints, concerns over quality of patient care, patient expectations, new and innovative technologies, legal limitations, and public opinion. This article discusses the current state of general surgery resident autonomy, why autonomy is important, barriers to autonomy, and ways to support autonomy.

**Early Detection and Remediation of Problem Learners**        611

Lilah F. Morris-Wiseman and Valentine N. Nfonsam

There are myriad types of problem learners in surgical residency and most have difficulty in more than 1 competency. Programs that use a standard curriculum of study and assessment are most successful in identifying struggling learners early. Many problem learners lack appropriate systems for study; a multidisciplinary educational team that is separate from the team that evaluates the success of remediation is critical. Struggling residents who require formal remediation benefit from performance improvement plans that clearly outline the issues of concern, describe the steps required for remediation, define success of remediation, and outline consequences for failure to remediate appropriately.

**Maintaining Wellness and Instilling Resilience in General Surgeons**    625

Jessica Brittany Weiss, Michael Minh Vu, Quinton Morrow Hatch, and Vance Young Sohn

Fostering wellness and enhancing resilience wellness and enhancing resilience will be increasingly more important for General Surgeons. Although these concepts are not new, the increased complexity of health care delivery has elevated the importance of these essential attributes. Instilling these practices should be emphasized during surgery residency and be modeled by surgical educators and surgeon leaders. The enhanced emphasis of wellness and resiliency is a positive step forward; however, more must be accomplished to ensure the well-being of a particularly group of vulnerable physicians. This chapter discusses the history and scientific theory behind wellness and resiliency, as well as practical suggestions for consideration.

**Medical Student Selection**    635

Ian Kratzke, Muneera R. Kapadia, Fumiko Egawa, and Jennifer S. Beaty

Medical school admissions committees are tasked with fulfilling the values of their institutions through careful recruitment. Making accurate predictions regarding the enrollment behavior of admitted students is critical to intentionally formulating class composition and impacts long-term physician representation.

**Attracting the Best Students to a Surgical Career**    653

Cameron St. Hilaire, Tatyana Kopilova, and Jeffrey M. Gauvin

The predicted shortage of surgeons in the future workforce is already occurring in rural areas and is expected to worsen. US allopathic medical school graduates have been losing interest in surgery for the past 40 years. The residency match remains unaffected because of foreign and osteopathic applicants. Negative myths regarding surgeon training, lifestyle, and personality persist among medical students, proving to be a powerful deterrent to students who might consider a surgical career. Proven strategies for making surgery more attractive to students are not always used and can be as simple as getting early exposure to students before clinical rotations.

**Evidence-Based Selection of Surgical Residents**    667

Laurel A. Vaughan and Jacob A. Quick

Residency programs should use a systematic method of recruitment that begins with defining unique desired candidate attributes. Commonly sought-after characteristics may be delineated via the residency application. Scores from standardized examinations taken in medical school predict academic success, and may correlate to overall performance. Strong letters of recommendation and a personal history of prior success outside the medical field both forecast success in residency. Interviews are crucial to determining fit within a program, and remain a valid measure of an applicant's ability to prosper in a particular program, even with many interviews being completed in the virtual realm.

## Value of Standardized Testing in Surgical Training                    679

Amy Han, Judith French, and Jeremy Lipman

Standardized testing remains a cornerstone of assessment in surgical education. Summative standardized tests make up a bulk of the certification requirements that encompasses demonstration of efficient, safe application of clinically relevant surgical knowledge and skills. Formative standardized tests serve similar role to guide teaching endeavors for the programs and comparison of individual trainees on a national level. Ongoing rigorous psychometric evaluations of the standardized tests ensure reliability and validity; however, standardized tests are not without their limitations and biases.

## Integration of Educational Technology                    693

Aditi Jalla, Jourdan Sturges, and Jason Lees

Continued advancement has forced medical education to accept new ways in which to incorporate technology into its curriculum. As a result, technology has become a cornerstone to all levels of the medical education. This article compiles and discusses various avenues in which technology serves and betters education, ranging from administrative databases to cloud-based storage. Overall, technology can serve various educational purposes, including compilation, circulation, and integration of educational materials. The modalities discussed within this article, while numerous and adaptable, are a small portion of what the technological world has to offer.

## Continuing Medical Education and Lifelong Learning                    703

Callie D. McAdams and Michael M. McNally

Continuing medical education is an ongoing process to educate clinicians and provide patients with up-to-date, evidence-based care. Since its inception, the maintenance of certification (MOC) program has changed dramatically. This article reviews the development of MOC and its integration with the 6 core competencies, including the practice-based learning and improvement cycle. The concept of lifelong learning is discussed, with specific focus on different methods for surgeons to engage in learning, including simulation, coaching, and communities of practice. In addition, the future of MOC in continuous professional development is reviewed.

# SURGICAL CLINICS
# OF NORTH AMERICA

**FORTHCOMING ISSUES**

*October 2021*
**Postoperative Complications**
Amy L. Lightner and Phillip Fleshner,
*Editors*

*December 2021*
**Controversies in General Surgery**
Sean J. Langenfeld, *Editor*

*February 2022*
**Surgical Critical Care**
Brett H. Waibel, *Editor*

**RECENT ISSUES**

*June 2021*
**Management of Esophageal Cancer**
John A. Federico, Thomas Fabian, *Editors*

*April 2021*
**Emerging Bariatric Surgical Procedures**
Shanu N. Kothari, *Editor*

*February 2021*
**Patient Safety**
Feibi Zheng, *Editor*

# SURGICAL CLINICS
# OF NORTH AMERICA

**FORTHCOMING ISSUES**

October 2021
Postoperative Complications
Amy L. Lightner and Phillip Fleshner,
Editors

December 2021
Controversies in General Surgery
Sean J. Langenfeld, Editor

February 2022
Surgical Critical Care
Kevin H. Wood, Editor

**RECENT ISSUES**

June 2021
Management of Esophageal Cancer
John A. Federico, Thomas Fabian, Editors

April 2021
Emergency Bedside Surgical Procedures
Shanu N. Kothari, Editor

February 2021
Nutrition Surgery
John J. Cheng, Editor

**SERIES OF RELATED INTEREST**

Advances in Surgery
http://www.advancessurgery.com/
Surgical Oncology Clinics
http://www.surgonc.theclinics.com/
Thoracic Surgery Clinics
http://www.thoracic.theclinics.com/

# Foreword

# Surgical Education

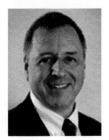

Ronald F. Martin, MD, FACS
*Consulting Editor*

*Prepare the child for the road, not the road for the child.*

*—Unknown*

I can think of few other endeavors in our surgical world that generate as much universal interest as the process of surgical education. After all, we all have been through it. Some of us make the process of formal education a large part of our day-to-day life, while others encounter education in small groups or perhaps even alone. Some are close to their medical school and residency training, while others remember their undergraduate and graduate medical training as distant memories. I have found though that no matter where a surgeon resides on the arc of her/his career development, she/he always has an opinion on how we *should* train learners and on whether learners are actually learning what they *need* to know.

In the realm of surgical education, we place extreme emphasis on training that occurs during surgical residency. Perhaps that is sensible in some regard. However, it may be possible that focusing on training in such a narrow way is forcing us to miss one of the real challenges of surgical education: it is difficult to state when learning to be a surgeon begins, and it even harder to state when it ends—it never really ends. For many years, surgical residency programs (and their collective directorships) have been lamenting the quality and quantity of training that medical school graduates have secured prior to their entry into residency programs. Many changes within medical schools and residencies have been attempted to try to mitigate those concerns with various degrees of success.

On the far side of residency training, both employers and fellowship directors have expressed their concerns about the completeness of training of those who have completed surgical residency programs. The overwhelming majority of graduates from standard general surgery residency programs now go on to some form of fellowship training: many to pursue focused studies in subspecialty

Surg Clin N Am 101 (2021) xiii–xv
https://doi.org/10.1016/j.suc.2021.05.023
0039-6109/21/© 2021 Published by Elsevier Inc.

areas, but many choose additional training to mitigate a perceived lack of comfort in surgical areas that historically were considered well covered with the core residency.

I submit that we largely focus on education during the period of medical school though residency and fellowship because they are time based. It makes for an easy target to allege that training begins at $x$ and ends at $y$. The fact that these intervals do follow specific time frames is not because they naturally lend themselves to it, but possibly is more reflective of the reality of how "training" is monetized: students pay tuition for medical school and residents and/or fellows are paid for with partially or completely subsidized funds from some other source than their employer—usually the federal government (at least in the United States).

To me, this is where the "time-based" concept of training always breaks down. It seems intuitive enough that it should never have to be stated, but surgical education—like all other education—begins with everything one has learned and never really ends.

After formal graduate medical education, we espouse concepts such as professional development, self-assessment, continuing medical education, maintenance of competence (or certification), or any other term of art that all refer to the same basic concept—we need to keep learning. Though one could argue that we all don't need to keep learning the same things. There are certain "building blocks" that any given practicing surgeon will need to know to safely care for patients within a designated scope of clinical problems. That said, there is probably far more variability than commonality in what any given surgeon will need demonstrable facility in depending on the environment in which she works or the collective skills of the colleagues with whom she works. Whether one works in a tertiary/quaternary referral center or a small hospital that is a helicopter's ride away from its nearest neighbor facility likely has more impact on what we need to stay current with educationally than our more standardized training model may suggest.

We all need to learn, and we all need to teach. We need to teach ourselves, our colleagues, our patients, and our communities. In the quote above, we all are the child who is trying to prepare for the road. Grown up and adult as we all may be, we are still the neophyte who is trying to learn how to navigate the next step of our career or our life—even if the next step is knowing when to stop. While we all wish to make the path easier to travel for those who follow us, we must always remember to teach those behind us how to maintain the roads they have inherited and create their own paths to improve as well.

Our Guest Editor, Dr P.J. Schenarts, and I have been walking this path of surgical education on the same roads or parallel roads for most of our surgical careers. We have spent many hours agreeing and disagreeing on how best to make the journey—mostly agreeing. We at the *Surgical Clinics* are deeply indebted to him and his colleagues, who have put together a comprehensive and insightful set of articles to help us understand how we learn and how we may be better able to teach. I think no matter where or how you practice, or how close you are to the beginning or the later stages of your surgical career, this information will be of enormous help to you.

As you consider this material, I urge you to ask yourself if you could be a better learner and a better teacher. It may be a challenge to consider this for many of us. It is for me. One lesson that I hope I have learned is that as a learner I would benefit to better adjust myself to the ways of my teachers. That has been hard to do; yet not as hard as realizing that as a teacher I need to better adjust how I teach to the ways of the learners. No matter my view of how learning and teaching should be done or the view of the learner as to the better way, the simple truth lies in that learning and teaching are inherently bidirectional in nature and do not exist well as monopolar concepts. We may all need to find a way stay in the center of the road and avoid navigating by bouncing off the guardrails of life.

Ronald F. Martin, MD, FACS
Colonel (retired), United States Army Reserve
Department of General Surgery and
Surgical Oncology
Madigan Army Medical Center
9040 Jackson Avenue
Tacoma, WA 98431, USA

*E-mail address:*
rfmcescna@gmail.com

# Preface

# Surgical Education

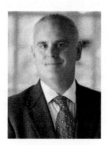

Paul J. Schenarts, MD, FACS
*Editor*

*Since my house burnt down, I now have a better view of the rising moon.*
—*Mizuta Masahide, Seventeenth Century Samurai[1]*

The COVID-19 pandemic has had a transformational effect on surgical education. The impact has been experienced globally, across all specialties and at all educational levels. The rise of virtual learning platforms was a necessary response but only a fair replacement for live educational conferences and a poor substitute for actual clinical experience. The reduction of patients seeking care for non-COVID illnesses, decreased number of nonemergency operations, fewer outpatient experiences, and redeployment of the surgical workforce to nonsurgical areas may negatively impact surgeons and their patients for years to come.

Under these conditions, the goal of preparing medical students for entry into residency and residents for fellowship or practice, while not lowering standards, is a righteous one, righteous yet unattainable without a renewed focus on the basic elements of education. The genesis of this issue of *Surgical Clinics* occurred at the start of the pandemic. As such, the focus was not on the educational impact of this disease but rather on providing a comprehensive review across the full educational lifecycle of a surgeon. Like in many aspects of medicine, serendipity favors the prepared. As we begin to navigate past the immediate crisis of the pandemic, surgeons will have to educationally compensate for potential shortcomings and lack of experiences for their medical students, residents, and junior partners. The purpose of this issue is to provide a comprehensive, up-to-date, and practical resource for all those who prepare the surgeons of tomorrow.

This issue of *Surgical Clinics* focuses on 4 major areas in surgical education. It begins with the biology of how we learn the factual and technical aspects of surgery, followed by how we select students who will be successful in medical school, and then how to attract the best students to a surgical career. Attention is then turned toward

https://doi.org/10.1016/j.suc.2021.05.022
0039-6109/21/© 2021 Published by Elsevier Inc.
surgical.theclinics.com

residency training with articles on evidenced-based selection of surgical residents, early detection, and remediation of the problem learner. The third area of focus is on effective teachings skills. This section addresses teaching in small groups and large lecture halls as well as technical and nontechnical skills. The integration of advanced technology into education and the value of standardized testing are also addressed. The final area of focus is the transition from resident into practice and beyond. This transition begins with a comprehensive review of the facts and myths about learner autonomy. Lifelong learning as well as maintaining wellness and instilling resilience closes out this issue.

This issue of *Surgical Clinics* was written during the height of the pandemic storm. Several of the authors and close family members of others were infected by COVID-19. Some experienced the deaths of surgical partners and friends. All had to guide their own trainees through the clinical and emotional aspects of this terrible crisis. I will be forever indebted to each author for their steadfast commitment and flexibility in completion of this work.

Paul J. Schenarts, MD, FACS
Des Moines University
College of Osteopathic Medicine
3200 Grand Avenue
Des Moines, IA 50312-4198, USA

Creighton University
School of Medicine
Omaha, NE, USA

*E-mail addresses:*
paul.schenarts@dmu.edu; pjschenartsmd@gmail.com

**REFERENCE**

1. Available at: https://www.inspiringquotes.us/author/3408-miztua-masahide. Accessed on March 5, 2021.

# The Biology and Psychology of Surgical Learning

Paul J. Schenarts, MD[a,b,*], Rachel E. Schenkel, MD[a], Maura E. Sullivan, PhD[c]

## KEYWORDS

- Surgical education • Surgical training • Learning • Memory
- Educational psychology

## KEY POINTS

- A scientific understanding of learning can be applied to surgical education.
- Biologic and psychological elements intertwine to influence learning.
- Environmental factors relevant to surgical training can interfere with effective learning.
- Certain teaching techniques can optimize information absorption, understanding, and recall.

*Change is the end result of true learning.*

—*Leo Buscaglia[1]*

A surgeon's knowledge and technical skills are not innate, but rather learned. Although different branches of neuroscience and psychology use slightly different definitions,[2–4] at its root, learning is the biological process of acquiring new knowledge by forming associations between different stimuli in our environment. Memory is the process of retaining and reconstructing that knowledge over time[2] and allows us to translate these associations into behavioral change.[3]

In biophysiological terms, learning is the rewiring of a plastic or dynamic nervous system owing to experiences and memory residing in this changed wiring.[3] Although scientific advances support this hypothesis, the concept is ancient. The philosopher Socrates considered memory to be like a wax tablet into which memories were imprinted; if the wax was too hard or if these impressions were rubbed out, we would not remember or learn.[5]

This article presents a concise conceptual framework of learning that begins with the biology of neuronal connections and the brain. The second section focuses on

[a] Departments of Surgery, Creighton University, School of Medicine, Creighton University Education Building, Suite 501, 7710 Mercy Road, Omaha, NE 68124-2368, USA; [b] Des Moines University; [c] Department of Surgery, University of Southern California, Los Angeles, CA 90033, USA
* Corresponding author. Professor, Department of Surgery, Creighton University, School of Medicine, Creighton University Education Building, Suite 501, 7710 Mercy Road, Omaha, NE 68124-2368, USA.
*E-mail address:* paulschenarts@creighton.edu

Surg Clin N Am 101 (2021) 541–554
https://doi.org/10.1016/j.suc.2021.05.002
0039-6109/21/© 2021 Elsevier Inc. All rights reserved.
surgical.theclinics.com

the psychology of learning, including the importance of cognitive load, knowledge retrieval, and adult learning. The article concludes with a return to the cellular level, where we discuss other factors that influence memory, learning, and skill acquisition, including stress,[6–8] sleep,[8–10] and unconscious bias,[11] all of which have a biologic basis. It is unreasonable to attempt to provide an exhaustive review of such complex biological and psychological processes in a single article. Therefore, our approach is selectively concise and provides a foundation for the articles that follow.

## THE NEUROANATOMY AND NEUROPHYSIOLOGY OF MEMORY AND LEARNING

Memory is the fundamental component of learning. Although each has different definitions, the mechanisms of learning cannot be separated from memory expression.[3]

The idea that specific brain functions are localized to distinct areas of the brain was well-established by the early nineteenth century.[12] A combination of observations of traumatically injured patients and results of experimentally induced lesions produced strikingly specific effects, including selective memory impairment.[12–14] Other early studies also suggested that memory is distributed throughout the cortex.[12,15] Based on more advanced study, including the use of functional MRI, positron emission tomography, and genetically altered knockout mice, the modern interpretation is that memory is indeed distributed, but that different anatomic areas store different features of the whole.[16]

## TYPES OF MEMORY

Memory is generally categorized by the time over which it is effective. The first category is immediate memory or sensory memory. This type of memory is effective within fractions of a second and is basically the brain's ability to hold onto an ongoing experience. All new information enters our cognition via the sensory memory. Both visual and auditory systems perceive a vast number of incoming stimuli and hold any given piece of information for only a brief period. These primarily sensory experiences are almost immediately forgotten[17] and do not reach conscious awareness unless they specifically catch our attention, such as, seeing a familiar face among dozens of people in a crowd. In other words, our attention allows us to "screen out" irrelevant stimuli and "screen in" relevant words and images.[18]

Once we attend to information in sensory memory, the information moves to the next temporal category, which is short-term or working memory. This memory allows us to hold and manipulate information for seconds to minutes while it is being used to achieve a specific goal. The most important thing to understand about the working memory is that it has a very limited[19] capacity and is only able to retain $7 \pm 2$ elements of information at any given time.[19] Almost all information in the working memory is lost within seconds if it is not refreshed by active rehearsal (eg, repeating to oneself a phone number or laboratory value). As such, short-term memory is pertinent to language, reasoning, and problem solving.[17] It is the short-term memory that is impacted most negatively by distraction.

The third category is long-term memory. Information of significance in immediate or short-term memory may enter the long-term memory by conscious or unconscious rehearsal, where it connects with related stored knowledge and remains for days to a lifetime.[17] Information can be held indefinitely in the long-term memory and this feature allows us the ability to store and recall information for future use.[20]

## NEURONAL WIRING: THE ANATOMIC MANIFESTATION OF LEARNING

The transformation of immediate and short-term memories into long-term ones involves the electrophysiologic strengthening of specific neuronal connections and the weakening of others.[17,21–23] The activated N-methyl-D-aspartate receptors and various intracellular signals that originate in the postsynaptic membranes can promote the synthesis of new proteins and the dynamics of actin. The consecutive morphologic changes in the cytoskeleton of the neuron, later stabilized by new receptors inserted in the postsynaptic membranes, make possible memory consolidation.[2,24,25] In short, neurons that fire together will wire together.

The notion that memory was due to strengthening neuronal connections was proposed more than 125 years ago by the Spanish neuroanatomist Santiago Ramon y Caja.[26] At that time, the (since disproven) dogma was that the adult brain could not grow new neurons. Therefore, it was a reasonable assumption that the key changes in storage and retrieval of new memories must occur between already existing neurons.[21] Although the reasoning for this assumption was incorrect, it has since been accepted that the chemical synapses of the brain are capable of undergoing plastic changes that either strengthen or weaken synaptic transmission.[22,23] This short-term synaptic plasticity lasts minutes, but long-term plasticity in the brain also exists. This process requires protein synthesis and genetic expression to construct new synapses and new, enlarged dendritic spines.[2,17,21] In other words, the collection of these new and strengthened neural connections into a memory is the physical manifestation of learning, termed an engram.[27,28]

These physical changes to the neurons of the hippocampus are further stabilized by the process of consolidation, which also involves genetic expression and protein synthesis. Although these electrophysiologic and anatomic changes to the structures of the medial temporal lobe are important in memory acquisition, they last only a few weeks, which is enough time for the consolidation of these memories in various areas of the neocortex, where they are ultimately stored.[3,16,23]

## ANATOMY AND PHYSIOLOGY OF MEMORY RETRIEVAL

The retrieval or reactivation of a memory is a complex process. In addition to the medial temporal lobe, other structures also support the initial perception, processing, and long-term storage of the experience. A long-standing view is that the cortical processing of a multisensory experience leaves a distributed record in the same multiple regions that initially performed the processing. For example, neurons in visual areas store the visual aspect of a multisensory experience, neurons in auditory areas store the auditory aspect of the experience, other areas store the spatial aspects, and so on. According to this view, any act of remembering consists of the coordinated reactivation of the distributed neocortical regions that were engaged at the time of encoding.[29–32] When a memory is first formed, this reactivation depends on the hippocampus and related structures, but once a memory is fully consolidated, reactivation can occur independently in the neocortex.[16]

Although these chemical and physical adjustments account for changes in memory, anatomic location varies depending on the type of memory; explicit (declarative) memory for recall of facts, places, objects, and events versus implicit (nondeclarative) memory for perceptual or motor skills. In humans, explicit memory requires conscious awareness and is located anatomically primarily in the hippocampus and adjacent cortex.[2] The central role of the medial temporal lobe, the hippocampus, and adjacent cortex in memory have become well-known as the result of multiple publications about patients[33,34] with injuries in these specific areas[13,16,35,36] and is supported by several reports that hippocampal volume is typically decreased by 40% to 45% in patients who have sustained memory loss after an anoxic insult.[37,38]

Interestingly, although patients with injuries to the hippocampus had memory and factual learning difficulty, their abilities to learn eye–hand coordination tasks were preserved. This finding led to the realization that there must be another type of memory system. As opposed to explicit memory, implicit memory involves learning skills and does not require conscious awareness. This type of memory is localized to the cerebellum, the striatum, and the amygdala.[2,24,39] Further, the neostriatum (not the medial temporal lobe) is important for the sort of gradual, feedback-guided learning that results in habit memory.[33,34]

The learning of eye–hand coordination skills does not only involve increasing synaptic efficacy. In the cerebellum, the combined activation of 2 different synaptic inputs to a Purkinje neuron depresses the transmission efficacy at a synapse. This depression is persistent and is called long-term depression.[40,41] Long-term depression in the cerebellum is considered to be the cellular basis of motor learning.[42]

## OBSERVATIONAL LEARNING AND FUTURE RESEARCH

It is obvious that surgical education would require both explicit and implicit memory. However, much learning is observational in the early development of surgeons. Can the time spent observing surgical procedures be physiologically justified? As it turns out, adult brains have special mirror neurons that help us to compare an observed activity visually with a remembered action in our memory, an ability that helps us to imitate and learn through watching.[43]

Although there is consensus about the anatomic locations and electrophysiologic and biostructural changes that result in memory and learning, the pathways that allow entry into the hippocampus and eventual exit to the neocortex are not yet known. Further, the hypothesis outlined elsewhere in this article does not explain other important areas of memory and learning, such as how we use acquired information to move in space, construct frames of reference, or in contingency thinking.[2,3]

Although the concepts of neuroanatomy, synaptic biology, and the process of memory consolidation provide the physiologic foundation of learning, surgical education also depends on understanding the more pragmatic importance of educational psychology. The psychological aspects of how knowledge is organized, rehearsed, and retrieved, as well as the important concepts of motivation, relevance, and feedback, are uniquely important to the surgical educator.

## INFORMATION PROCESSING AND COGNITIVE LOAD

As mentioned elsewhere in this article, new information comes into our awareness through the sensory memory. Once something catches our attention, it is moved into the working memory where it must be attended to for it to become stored in the long-term memory. Owing to the limited capacity of the working memory, learning is impacted because many learning tasks require the processing of more than 7 units of information at a given time.[19] Otherwise known as the "bottleneck" of learning, the working memory is limited in both capacity and duration.[44] Learning is impaired when novel information or learning new tasks creates a cognitive load that exceeds the capacity of the working memory. Cognitive load theory, first described by Sweller in 1988,[45] focuses on the role of the working memory in learning[45] and helps us to understand how and why learners struggle with mastering complex content and developing expertise. According to cognitive load theory, there are 3 types of cognitive load that affect learning: intrinsic, extraneous, and germane. The intrinsic load is the cognitive demand associated with the task. It is the direct function of the complexity of the task and the experience of the learner. The greater the complexity of the information, the greater the intrinsic load of the task. The extraneous load refers to the cognitive energy that is consumed by factors that are not related to learning the task, such as distractions and ineffective teaching techniques. The germane load refers to the mental effort required for the learner to perform a task.[46] It is regulated by the individual and is the amount of effort or concentration devoted to the task.[44] When the extraneous and/or intrinsic loads exceed the limits of the working memory, there will be insufficient resources available for the germane load necessary for learning.[44]

There are specific strategies that can be used by faculty teachers to decrease the cognitive load theory of trainees. Intrinsic load can be decreased by simplifying information and providing preparatory training before the task. Extraneous load can be decreased by minimizing distractions and by presenting new information in an organized manner. Intrinsic and extrinsic loads are additive in nature. The extraneous load interferes with learning only if the intrinsic load for the task is high (ie, the task is difficult for the learner). When the intrinsic load associated with the task is low (ie, the task is easy), the extraneous load may not harm learning if the total load remains within the trainee's limitations.[47]

The complexity and urgency of the surgical training environment has the potential to produce cognitive overload for learners. When the number of informational elements exceeds working memory capacity, new information cannot be processed. This factor limits the learning and performance of the trainee. For the learner to work within these constraints, the working memory attempts to combine and organize new information into meaningful "chunks" or schema (plural schemata). A schema is an organized cognitive structure of knowledge or chunk of information. It attempts to organize multiple elements of information into a single representation according to how those elements relate to each other and how they will be stored in the long-term memory for future use.[20] Almost all information in the working memory is lost within seconds if it is not refreshed by active rehearsal strategies that help with storage and retrieval.

## KNOWLEDGE RETRIEVAL

To facilitate learning, students must retain the information they have encountered, relate novel information to other stored knowledge, and organize it in such a manner that it can be retrieved easily from the long-term memory for future use. Knowledge retrieval is enhanced when the following learning techniques are used and practiced: elaborative interrogation, self-explanation, summarization, and keyword mnemonics.

### Elaborative Interrogation

Elaborative interrogation is the process of generating an explanation for why information is true. As humans, we are inquisitive by nature and seek explanations for things around us. Research has shown that prompting learners to answer the question "why" material is important or true will promote knowledge understanding and help to organize new information.[48] This process is achieved by activating schema, which enhances learning by supporting the integration of new information with existing prior knowledge.[48]

### Self-Explanation

Self-explanation involves explaining how new information relates to previously learned knowledge or an explanation of steps taken during problem solving. Like elaborative interrogation, self-explanation may enhance learning by supporting the integration of new information with existing prior knowledge and organizing knowledge into schema for storage in the long-term memory.[48]

### Summarization

Summarization involves writing out important concepts in one's own words. Writing a summary of information helps learners to identify what is important, synthesize information, and understand how different ideas connect to one another. Summarization boosts learning and retention because it involves attending to and extracting higher level meaning. This process goes beyond merely selecting important information and has been shown to boost organizational processing.[48]

### Keyword Mnemonics

Keyword mnemonics are an elaborative rehearsal strategy based on interactive imagery. In this process, the learner forms a mental image of the keyword being connected to new information. Doing so helps to encode information more effectively so that information is more easily memorized and recalled. The mental images are the "cues" that help the brain to retrieve information more easily from the long-term memory. There is evidence that keyword mnemonics can boost memory for many kinds of material, which has made it a relatively popular technique.[49]

### ADULT TEACHING AND LEARNING

Many learning theories have been incorporated into medical education, a comprehensive review of which is beyond the scope of this article. Instead, we have chosen several foundational principles of teaching and learning from various theories that we feel provide the best foundation for medical educational programs. Here we propose 5 characteristics of teaching and learning that most impact adult learning: (1) active engagement, (2) content relevance, (3) motivation, (4) self-directed learning, and (5) feedback.

### Active Engagement

To maintain attention and promote learning and retention, students need to be engaged actively in the learning process. Active engagement is linked to experiential learning, which was first championed in the 1970s by David Kolb.[50] This theory postulates that adults are active constructors of learning and are shaped by their experiences. The best learning comes from making sense of your experiences and linking it to prior knowledge. Instead of memorizing facts and figures, experiential learning is a hands-on and reflective learning style approach.

### Content Relevance

Learning occurs best when the material is meaningful to the learner and is related to their real-world problems and experiences. Without seeing the relevance of materials, learners have difficulty applying it effectively to their own situation. A challenge for educators is to create an environment where students can find meaning in the content taught. This goal can often be achieved by sharing personal experiences and/or developing case scenarios to place the material into meaningful context.

### Motivation

One of the most important principles of adult learning is that the student is motivated to learn new information and attend to a task. Motivation reflects the desire to work toward a goal and helps to engage, direct, and sustain behavior.[51] Motivation enhances cognitive processing and leads to improved performance.[51] There are 2 types of motivation that we see in medical education: intrinsic and extrinsic. Intrinsic motivation is the desire to perform a goal based on an internal drive. For example, a student may be working to perform their personal best or may be working tirelessly owing to personal interest in a topic. Extrinsic motivation is when motivation comes from external forces, such as studying for an examination to get a good grade or hoping for a promotion. An effective faculty member can help students to increase intrinsic motivation by establishing content relevance and helping them to discover the need to learn subject material within themselves.

### Self-Directedness

Self-directed learning is the process where individuals take the initiative to diagnose their own learning needs, formulate learning goals, select resources and materials for learning, and evaluate their own learning outcomes.[52] Faculty members can help students to focus self-directed learning by helping them to identify gaps in their knowledge and set specific learning goals. The communication of learning goals between the learner and faculty member enhances student learning. Self-directed learning may also happen outside the clinical environment, with learners working either by themselves or as part of a self-directed learning process.

### Feedback

Feedback is the process of providing students with information about their performance as compared with a given standard with the goal of improving the student's overall performance. Learning effectiveness depends on feedback and it is one of the most critical requirements for learning.[53] Feedback has been shown to accelerate learning and help learners to achieve their goals.[53] Without feedback, mistakes can go uncorrected, learners may make inaccurate assumptions about their learning, and competency can be delayed.

Feedback should be specific and should focus on behaviors that the learners have the power to change. For example, telling a resident that they have poor operative skills because their hands are too big is not effective or reasonable; the aim should be to give the learner a more accurate description of what they should do differently. In addition, feedback should be given in a supportive environment and should be an interactive discussion between the faculty member and the learner. A good approach is to first ask the learner how things are going or what they think they should do differently. Usually, the learner can self-reflect and identify areas to focus on for improvement. This assessment can serve as a starting point for a feedback conversation. Constructive feedback conveys an attitude of concern regarding progress of the resident and, if done correctly, is valued by most learners.

In addition to the basic neurophysiologic and psychological aspects of surgical education, several other influences on memory and learning have come into greater focus. The impact of sleep and stress on learning has led to significant regulatory changes for surgical training programs.[54] More recently, the importance of implicit bias has been recognized among surgical educators, professional societies, and administrators.[55–59] The final section of this article examines to what extent each of these areas of concern has a biological foundation.

## IMPACT OF SLEEP ON THE BIOPHYSIOLOGY OF MEMORY AND LEARNING

There has probably been nothing more controversial over the past 20 years than the debate about the role of sleep deprivation and medical education. Searching the phrase "Sleep and surgical education" on PUBMED yields more than1200 citations.[60] Excluding sleep's impact on resident well-being, patient safety, and quality of education, what are the biophysiologic effects of sleep? Although the function of sleep remains largely unknown, several hypotheses have been proposed, including brain thermoregulation, detoxification, and tissue restoration. Another hypothesis is that periods of sleep are required for the brain plasticity required for learning and memory.[8–10]

The task of sorting out the interaction of sleep with memory is a dauntingly complex but is nicely summarized by the works of Walker[61] and Dickelmann and associates.[62,63] There is evolving and compelling evidence that sleep promotes long-term consolidation of explicit (facts) memories by synchronizing information transfer from the hippocampus, where memories are created, to the neocortex, where memories are stored and reactivated.[64,65] The conventional view is that the initial memory trace on neuronal pathway connections are fragile until the first postexposure sleep period.[8] Then, the slow oscillations of brain electrical activity during non-REM sleep enhances the neuronal activity in those neurons, which have recently undergone plastic synaptic change, thereby forming tighter connections between these neurons.[66,67] These slow wave oscillations also increase local gene activity required for protein synthesis and structural neuronal change needed for long-term memory.[10,63]

Despite these accumulating data on the importance of sleep in forming explicit memories, the role of sleep in the acquisition or execution of physical skills is the subject of ongoing debate. It may be that sleep is required primarily when learning a sequence of steps or generating a new routine of physical movements.[65,68]

In conclusion, there is a neurophysiologic role for sleep in the establishment of long-term memory. However, there is no empiric evidence that current Accreditation Council for Graduate Medical Education duty-hour regulations[54] are in alignment with these molecular–biologic changes.

## IMPACT OF STRESS ON THE BIOPHYSIOLOGY OF MEMORY AND LEARNING

Like the controversy over the importance of sleep during training, the role of stress in education is a hot topic. In the book, *The Coddling of the American Mind*,[69] Lukianoff and Haidt articulate the arguments for and against the well-intentioned removal of stress from the learning environment. From a neurobiology standpoint, acute stress may favor memory formation and enhance learning.[70] Alternatively, too much stress has been shown to impair learning.[7]

The appraisal of a situation as stressful is highly subjective and made by the prefrontal cortex and limbic structures, especially the hippocampus and the amygdala, which link the current situation to experiences from the individuals' past. These brain regions relate to the hypothalamus, a central hub in the coordination of the physiologic response to stress. Within seconds after a stressful event, the hypothalamus activates the autonomic nervous system, which triggers the release of adrenaline and noradrenaline from the adrenal medulla. At the same time, the hypothalamus initiates a slower hormone cascade along the hypothalamus–pituitary–adrenal axis. This cascade leads via intermediate steps to the release of glucocorticoids from the adrenal cortex. In addition to adrenaline, noradrenaline, and glucocorticoids, numerous other hormones, neuropeptides, and neurotransmitters are released in response to a stressor. Together these stress mediators help the organism to adapt to the stressor and to restore homeostasis.[7] The specific impact of glucocorticoids on memory and learning is amplitude dependent. Low amplitude stress improves memory, whereas an excessive amplitude significantly impairs it.[43]

Stress can be extrinsic, external to the task, or intrinsic, related to the task itself. The neural cell adhesion molecule (NCAM) is a cell adhesion macromolecule known to play a critical role in the development and plasticity of the nervous system. NCAM is critically involved in the mechanisms of learning and memory, and its expression levels are known to be highly susceptible to modulation by stress. Although available data are insufficient to conclude as to whether NCAM mediates extrinsic stress effects on learning and memory processes, there is evidence supporting a key mediating role for NCAM in the facilitation of memory consolidation induced by intrinsic stress.[6]

The timing of the stress in relation to the learning experience is also important. If the stress occurs right at the beginning or the end of the learning experience, before consolidation, the memory performance is enhanced, whereas stress too far before the learning experience or after consolidation has a negative effect.[43]

In summary, the impact of stress on memory and learning could best be described as a "Goldilocks situation." Too much or too little does not help learning and the amount and timing need to be just right. It should also be noted that previously learned responses can also be influenced by stress. Under stressful conditions, rigid habit memory is favored over more cognitive flexible memory.[7]

## THE BIOLOGY OF IMPLICIT BIAS

Implicit bias refers to the attitudes or stereotypes that affect our understanding, actions, and decisions in an unconscious manner. These biases, which encompass both favorable and unfavorable assessments, are activated involuntarily and without an individual's awareness or intentional control. Residing deep in the subconscious, these biases are different from known biases that individuals may choose to conceal for the purposes of social and/or political correctness.[71]

The dramatic impact of implicit bias (unconscious bias) in surgical education and surgical culture is coming into focus.[55–59] To provide a comprehensive overview of this important topic is well beyond the scope of this article. The biological basis for this process has been expertly reviewed by Reihl and colleagues[11] and Amodio and associates.[72,73]

From neurobiological and evolutionary standpoints, implicit bias in an unconscious process that helps us to differentiate or group people into an "in group" (those who are like us) from an "out group" (those who are different.) This neurobiological automatic reflex is based in the amygdala and is not under conscious control.[11,72–74] This fast process is in competition with the anatomically distinct areas of the brain responsible for the much slower process of high-order reasoning.[11,72–74] This dual system explains why a person may act in unintentional discriminatory fashion while articulating they believe the opposite.

There is an educational impact of unconsciously placing a learner in the "out group."

Implicit bias has been shown to influence medical school admissions,[56,75] surgery clerkship grades,[76] residency applications,[76–79] a diminished degree of operative autonomy,[80,81] and results in female presenters at national surgical meetings being informally introduced.[58]

There is also a large literature demonstrating the negatively influence of implicit bias on the quality of care certain patients receive.[82–84]

Because these automatic assessments of external stimuli are not under our control and are essential in a rapidly changing environment,[72–74] initial efforts to change behavior may be ineffective.[11] The Ohio State University, Kirwan Institute for the Study of Race and Ethnicity has been a pioneer in developing training modules for institutions and individuals[71] (https://kirwaninstitute.osu.edu). Recent educational literature is also demonstrating effective strategies against the negative influence of this unconscious biological phenomena.[55,85,86]

## SUMMARY

Surgical education requires proficiency with multiple types of learning to create capable surgeons. The complex relationships between the biological aspects of memory formation and the psychological aspects of data organization and recall all contribute to our ultimate grasp of a subject. In the world of surgical training, these factors are modulated by cognitive load, knowledge retrieval techniques, and adult learning. Factors such as stress, sleep, and unconscious bias also influence learning and memory and have been hot button issues in surgical training in recent years. The articles in this issue provide a more comprehensive examination of these topics.

## REFERENCES

1. Available at: https://www.brainyquote.com/quotes/leo_buscaglia_121067. Accessed December 15, 2020.
2. Kandel ER, Dudai Y, Mayford MR. The molecular and systems biology of memory. Cell 2014;157(1):163–86.
3. Gallistel CR, Matzel LD. The neuroscience of learning: beyond the Hebbian synapse. Annu Rev Psychol 2013;64:169–200.
4. Frankland PW, Josselyn SA, Köhler S. The neurobiological foundation of memory retrieval. Nat Neurosci 2019;22(10):1576–85.
5. Available at: https://www.historyofinformation.com/detail.php?id=3538. Accessed 15 December 2020.
6. Bisaz R, Conboy L, Sandi C. Learning under stress: a role for the neural cell adhesion molecule NCAM. Neurobiol Learn Mem 2009;91(4):333–42.
7. Schwabe L, Wolf OT, Oitzl MS. Memory formation under stress: quantity and quality. Neurosci Biobehav Rev 2010;34(4):584–91.
8. Maquet P. The role of sleep in learning and memory. Science 2001;294(5544): 1048–52.
9. Born J, Rasch B, Gais S. Sleep to remember. Neuroscientist 2006;12(5):410–24.
10. Dang-Vu TT, Desseilles M, Peigneux P, et al. A role for sleep in brain plasticity. Pediatr Rehabil 2006;9(2):98–118.
11. Reihl KM, Hurley RA, Taber KH. Neurobiology of implicit and explicit bias: implications for clinicians. J Neuropsychiatry Clin Neurosci 2015;27(4):A6–253.
12. Finger S. Origins of neuroscience: a history of explorations into brain function. New York: Oxford Univ. Press; 1994.
13. Scoville WB, Milner B. Loss of recent memory after bilateral hippocampal lesions. J Neurol Neurosurg Psychiatry 1957;20(1):11–21.
14. Penfield W, Milner B. Memory deficit produced by bilateral lesions in the hippocampal zone. AMA Arch Neurol Psychiatry 1958;79(5):475–97.
15. Lashley KS. Brain mechanisms and intelligence: a quantitative study of injuries to the brain. Chicago: Chicago Univ. Press; 1929.
16. Squire LR, Wixted JT. The cognitive neuroscience of human memory since H.M. Annu Rev Neurosci 2011;34:259–88.
17. Purves D, Augistine GJ, Fitzpatrick D, et al. Neuroscience. 6th ed. New York: Oxford University Press; 2018.
18. Mayer RE. Applying the science of learning to medical education. Med Educ 2010;44(6):543–9.
19. Miller GA. The magical number seven plus or minus two: some limits on our capacity for processing information. Psychol Rev 1956;63(2):81–97.

20. Gagne ED, Yekovich CW, Yekovich FR. The cognitive psychology of school learning. 2nd ed. New York, NY: Harper Collins College Publishers; 1993.
21. Miller G. How are memories stored and retrieved? Science 2005;309(5731):92.
22. Martin SJ, Grimwood PD, Morris RG. Synaptic plasticity and memory: an evaluation of the hypothesis. Annu Rev Neurosci 2000;23:649–711.
23. Martin SJ, Morris RG. New life in an old idea: the synaptic plasticity and memory hypothesis revisited. Hippocampus 2002;12(5):609–36.
24. Kandel ER. The molecular biology of memory storage: a dialog between genes and synapses. Biosci Rep 2004;24(4–5):475–522.
25. Morgado-Bernal I. Learning and memory consolidation: linking molecular and behavioral data. Neuroscience 2011;176:12–9.
26. Cajal SR. La fine structure des centres nerveux. The Croonian Lecture. Proc R Soc Lond 1894;55:444–68.
27. Tonegawa S, Pignatelli M, Roy DS, et al. Memory engram storage and retrieval. Curr Opin Neurobiol 2015;35:101–9.
28. Josselyn SA, Tonegawa S. Memory engrams: recalling the past and imagining the future. Science 2020;367(6473):eaaw4325.
29. Mishkin M. A memory system in the monkey. Philos Trans R Soc Lond B Biol Sci 1982;298(1089):83–95.
30. Zola-Morgan S, Squire LR, Mishkin M. The neuroanatomy of amnesia: amygdala-hippocampus versus temporal stem. Science 1982;218(4579):1337–9.
31. Squire LR, Shimamura AP, Graf P. Strength and duration of priming effects in normal subjects and amnesic patients. Neuropsychologia 1987;25(1B): 195–210.
32. Damasio AR. Time-locked multiregional retroactivation: a systems-level proposal for the neural substrates of recall and recognition. Cognition 1989; 33(1–2):25–62.
33. Murray EA, Mishkin M. Severe tactual as well as visual memory deficits follow combined removal of the amygdala and hippocampus in monkeys. J Neurosci 1984;4(10):2565–80.
34. Murray EA, Mishkin M. Relative contributions of SII and area 5 to tactile discrimination in monkeys. Behav Brain Res 1984;11(1):67–83.
35. Zola-Morgan S, Squire LR, Ramus SJ. Severity of memory impairment in monkeys as a function of locus and extent of damage within the medial temporal lobe memory system. Hippocampus 1994;4(4):483–95.
36. Rempel-Clower NL, Zola SM, Squire LR, et al. Three cases of enduring memory impairment after bilateral damage limited to the hippocampal formation. J Neurosci 1996;16(16):5233–55.
37. Cipolotti L, Shallice T, Chan D, Fox N, Scahill R, Harrison G, Stevens J, Rudge P. Long-term retrograde amnesia...the crucial role of the hippocampus. Neuropsychologia 2001;39(2):151–72.
38. Isaacs EB, Vargha-Khadem F, Watkins KE, et al. Developmental amnesia and its relationship to degree of hippocampal atrophy. Proc Natl Acad Sci U S A 2003; 100(22):13060–3.
39. Squire LR. Memory and the hippocampus: a synthesis from findings with rats, monkeys, and humans. Psychol Rev 1992;99(2):195–231.
40. Ito M, Sakurai M, Tongroach P. Climbing fibre induced depression of both mossy fibre responsiveness and glutamate sensitivity of cerebellar Purkinje cells. J Physiol 1982;324:113–34.
41. Ito M. Long-term depression. Annu Rev Neurosci 1989;12:85–102.

42. Okano H, Hirano T, Balaban E. Learning and memory. Proc Natl Acad Sci U S A 2000;97(23):12403–4.

43. Collins JW. The neuroscience of learning. J Neurosci Nurs 2007;39(5): 305–10.

44. Young JQ, Van Merrienboer J, Durning S, et al. Cognitive load theory: implications for medical education: AMEE Guide No. 86. Med Teach 2014;36(5): 371–84.

45. Sweller J. Cognitive load during problem solving: effects on learning. Cogn Sci 1988;12:257–85.

46. van Merriënboer JJ, Sweller J. Cognitive load theory in health professional education: design principles and strategies. Med Educ 2010;44(1):85–93.

47. Carlson R, Chandler P, Sweller J. Learning and understanding science instructional material. J Educ Psychol 2003;95:629–40.

48. Dunlosky J, Rawson KA, Marsh EJ, et al. Improving students' learning with effective learning techniques: promising directions from cognitive and educational psychology. Psychol Sci Public Interest 2013;14(1):4–58.

49. Hunt RR. The concept of distinctiveness in memory research. In: Hunt RR, Worthen JB, editors. Distinctiveness and memory. New York, NY: Oxford University Press; 2006. p. 3–25.

50. Kolb DA. Experiential learning: experience as the source of learning and development. Upper Saddle River, NJ: Prentice-Hall; 1984. p. 19–38.

51. Clark RE, Estes F. Turning research into results: a guide to selecting the right performance solutions. Atlanta, GA: CEP Press; 2002.

52. Knowles M, Holton E, Swanson R, editors. The adult learner: the definitive classic in adult education and human resource development. 8th Edition. New York, NY: Routledge; 2015.

53. Archer J. State of the science in health professional education: effective feedback. Med Education 2010;44:101–8.

54. Available at: https://www.acgme.org/Portals/0/PFAssets/ProgramRequirements/CPRResidency2020.pdf. Accessed December 15, 2020.

55. Backhus LM, Lui NS, Cooke DT, et al. Unconscious bias: addressing the hidden impact on surgical education. Thorac Surg Clin 2019;29(3):259–67.

56. Capers Q 4th, Clinchot D, McDougle L, et al. Implicit racial bias in medical school admissions. Acad Med 2017;92(3):365–9.

57. Dossa F, Baxter NN. Implicit bias in surgery-hiding in plain sight. JAMA Netw Open 2019;2(7):e196535.

58. Davids JS, Lyu HG, Hoang CM, et al. Female representation and implicit gender bias at the 2017 American Society of Colon and Rectal Surgeons' annual scientific and tripartite meeting. Dis Colon Rectum 2019;62(3):357–62.

59. Foster SM, Knight J, Velopulos CG, et al. Gender distribution and leadership trends in trauma surgery societies. Trauma Surg Acute Care Open 2020;5(1): e000433.

60. Available at: https://pubmed,ncbi.nih.gov/?term=sleep+and+surgical+education. Accessed December 15, 2020.

61. Walker MP, Stickgold R. Sleep-dependent learning and memory consolidation. Neuron 2004;44(1):121–33.

62. Diekelmann S, Wilhelm I, Born J. The whats and whens of sleep-dependent memory consolidation. Sleep Med Rev 2009;13(5):309–21.

63. Diekelmann S, Born J. The memory function of sleep. Nat Rev Neurosci 2010; 11(2):114–26.

64. Marshall L, Born J. The contribution of sleep to hippocampus-dependent memory consolidation. Trends Cogn Sci 2007;11(10):442–50.
65. Dudai Y, Karni A, Born J. The consolidation and transformation of memory. Neuron 2015;88(1):20–32.
66. Mölle M, Born J. Slow oscillations orchestrating fast oscillations and memory consolidation. Prog Brain Res 2011;193:93–110.
67. Born J. Slow-wave sleep and the consolidation of long-term memory. World J Biol Psychiatry 2010;11(Suppl 1):16–21.
68. Debas K, Carrier J, Barakat M, et al. Off-line consolidation of motor sequence learning results in greater integration within a cortico-striatal functional network. Neuroimage 2014;99:50–8.
69. Lukianoff G, Haidt J. The coddling of the American mind. Washington, DC: Penguin Random House; 2018.
70. Roozendaal B. 1999 Curt P. Richter award. Glucocorticoids and the regulation of memory consolidation. Psychoneuroendocrinology 2000;25(3):213–38.
71. Available at: http://kirwaninstitute.osu.edu/research/understanding-implicit-bias. Accessed December 15, 2020.
72. Amodio DM. The neuroscience of prejudice and stereotyping. Nat Rev Neurosci 2014;15(10):670–82.
73. Amodio DM, Cikara M. The social neuroscience of prejudice. Annu Rev Psychol 2020;72:439–69.
74. Shkurko AV. Is social categorization based on relational ingroup/outgroup opposition? A meta-analysis. Soc Cogn Affect Neurosci 2013;8(8):870–7.
75. Chatterjee A, Greif C, Witzburg R, et al. US Medical School applicant experiences of bias on the interview trail. J Health Care Poor Underserved 2020;31(1):185–200.
76. Chen S, Beck Dallaghan GL, Shaheen A. Implicit gender bias in third-year surgery clerkship MSPE narratives. J Surg Educ 2021;72:439–69.
77. Turrentine FE, Dreisbach CN, St Ivany AR, et al. Influence of gender on surgical residency applicants' recommendation letters. J Am Coll Surg 2019;228(4):356–65.e3.
78. Powers A, Gerull KM, Rothman R, et al. Race- and gender-based differences in descriptions of applicants in the letters of recommendation for orthopaedic surgery residency. JB JS Open Access 2020;5(3):e20.00023.
79. Belmont PJ Jr, Hoffmann JD, Tokish JM, et al. Overview of the military orthopaedic surgery residency application and selection process. Mil Med 2013;178(9):1016–23.
80. Meyerson SL, Odell DD, Zwischenberger JB, et al, Procedural Learning and Safety Collaborative. The effect of gender on operative autonomy in general surgery residents. Surgery 2019;166(5):738–43.
81. Joh DB, van der Werf B, Watson BJ, et al. Assessment of autonomy in operative procedures among female and male New Zealand general surgery trainees. JAMA Surg 2020;155(11):1019–26.
82. FitzGerald C, Hurst S. Implicit bias in healthcare professionals: a systematic review. BMC Med Ethics 2017;18(1):19.
83. Dehon E, Weiss N, Jones J, et al. A systematic review of the impact of physician implicit racial bias on clinical decision making. Acad Emerg Med 2017;24(8):895–904.
84. Green AR, Carney DR, Pallin DJ, et al. Implicit bias among physicians and its prediction of thrombolysis decisions for black and white patients. J Gen Intern Med 2007;22(9):1231–8.

85. Sherman MD, Ricco J, Nelson SC, et al. Implicit bias training in a residency program: aiming for enduring effects. Fam Med 2019;51(8):677–81.
86. Gonzalez CM, Garba RJ, Liguori A, et al. How to make or break implicit bias instruction: implications for curriculum development. Acad Med 2018. 93(11S Association of American Medical Colleges Learn Serve Lead: Proceedings of the 57th Annual Research in Medical Education Sessions):S74-S81.

# Teaching on Rounds and in Small Groups

Christopher Thomas, MD[a], Leah Plumblee, MD[a], Sean Dieffenbaugher, MD[b], Cynthia Talley, MD[a],*

## KEYWORDS

- Bedside teaching • Near-peer teaching • Residents • Attending preceptors
- Rounds • Small Groups

## KEY POINTS

- One-minute preceptor, Near-peer teaching, and structured bedside rounds lead to improved patient satisfaction and clinical skills in students and residents.
- There are several ways that surgical educators can better structure bedside rounds— pre-round preparation, set the scene, engage the patient, and the postround huddle.
- Problem-based and case-based learning as well as flipped classrooms facilitate small group learning in a supportive environment encouraging teamwork and creativity.

## TEACHING ON ROUNDS
### Background

When we think about teaching on rounds, we often reminisce about how we were taught during medical school. For many, this involved traditional bedside teaching in which a patient was presented to the attending surgeon and feedback was received on the assessment and plans for the patient. Effective teaching on rounds remains an evolving, often elusive process. This article highlights several popular methods, including bedside rounds, near-peer teaching, resident versus attending preceptors, and how teaching on rounds has an impact on patients. The 1-minute preceptor followed by an illustrative case is discussed.

Bedside teaching plays a vital role in the training of future physicians across all specialties. It is a method that allows for instruction in history taking, physical examination skills, differential diagnosis development, professionalism, teamwork integration, and effective communication and discussions of medical ethics. In the 1960s, bedside teaching comprised as much as 75% of all clinical training.[1] Unfortunately, due to the changes in the health care system, accreditation bodies, and shortened

[a] Medical University of South Carolina, Department of Surgery, 96 Jonathan Lucas Street, Charleston, SC 29425, USA; [b] Carolinas Medical Center, Atrium Health, Department of Surgery, 1000 Blythe Boulevard, MEB Office 601, Charlotte, NC 28203, USA
* Corresponding author. Medical University of South Carolina, Department of Surgery, 96 Jonathan Lucas Street, CSB 417D, MSC 613, Charleston, SC 29425.
E-mail address: talleyc@musc.edu

Surg Clin N Am 101 (2021) 555–563
https://doi.org/10.1016/j.suc.2021.05.003
0039-6109/21/© 2021 Elsevier Inc. All rights reserved.

admittance of patients, the rates of bedside teaching declined to 8% to 19% by the 2010s.[1] Attending surgeons are feeling increased external pressures to meet performance metrics while resident physicians must adhere to duty hour restrictions, raising the question of how to reincorporate bedside rounds in an efficient and meaningful way. As the father of modern medicine, Sir William Osler, stated regarding bedside teaching: "To study the phenomena of disease without books is to sail an uncharted sea, while to study without patients is not to go to sea at all."

### Barriers to Bedside Teaching Rounds

Five main barriers to bedside rounding include the following: factors related to the medical students, the timing of rounds, technological issues, the institution's view of the importance of bedside rounds, and the surgical educators' view of themselves as instructors. Although these issues can seem overwhelming, there are multiple ways to address them.

Medical school enrollment has increased steadily to meet the growing demand for physicians with the unfortunate consequence of increased numbers of students on surgery clerkships. This can have a direct negative effect on the quality of bedside teaching, with educators reporting difficulty being heard by all students.[2] Additionally, varying levels of learners during bedside rounds makes tailoring the topic and discussion more challenging. In the authors' experience, 1 of 2 options can help alleviate this issue: divide the student learners into smaller groups based on year of training, and tailor questions to student learner level with increasing difficulty for students or residents with more years of training.

Time constraints, faculty attitudes/knowledge, overreliance on technology, and learner autonomy are perceived barriers to effective bedside rounds according to learners.[3] Students excel when provided an in-person course orientation. The educator must provide the framework to engage the learner, express the metric for assessment, and provide timely feedback on completion of assigned responsibilities. Verbal reassurance by the attending physician lays the foundation for a positive learning environment. Students are more motivated to engage in educational activities if their surgical educator is able to provide them with adequate demonstration and guidance.[1,3]

Medical learners reported difficulty in remaining engaged during bedside rounds due to time factors—particularly when rounds lasted for a prolonged period of time or were conducted when the learner was post-call.[3] There is debate about the ideal timing for educational bedside rounds.[2–4] Although conducting teaching rounds in the early morning can disrupt the daily schedule and potentially have an impact on patient care activities (such as delayed discharges and delays in placing orders), many educators prefer this time because they view their team of learners to be more fresh and enthusiastic.[5] Other educators prefer to conduct bedside rounds in the afternoon, owing to better engagement of the learner because their clinical responsibilities can be accomplished earlier in the day with less distractions. One possible solution is to break rounds into manageable parts with a focused teaching time. Setting a firm day and time each week for educational bedside rounds allows other members of the multidisciplinary team to participate and minimize interruptions to the educational time.

As technology continues to improve the ability to diagnose and treat patients, some learners attribute the decrease in bedside teaching to this and question the utility of bedside physical examination of patients.[3] Many learners recognize that although technology has a time, place, and role in patient care, it cannot replace patient interactions. Technology's role within medical education continues to evolve. With increasing numbers of learners and educators having smart phones that can access a patient's electronic medical record, many people find themselves utilizing their devices during rounds. Many educators perceive that the learner is not participating in the discussion and care of the patient when accessing medical records by mobile device.[6] For this reason, it is important to set clear guidelines and expectations regarding the use of personal devices during bedside rounds with all participants at the start of rounds.

The culture within surgery departments can elevate the importance of bedside rounds and other educational opportunities. At many teaching hospitals, promotions are tied to publications and are minimally impacted by teaching evaluations with few to no ramifications for poor teaching evaluations. Those who excel in their bedside teaching evaluations should be celebrated because their efforts lead to direct improvements in learner test scores, satisfaction, and competence.[1,3,7] The educational institution should provide surgical educators with an integrated curriculum for bedside teaching and offer additional training to those educators who are struggling.[5]

Many surgical educators report a lack of confidence in their teaching abilities and anxiety related to bedside teaching.[2–5,7] Few residency programs offering development programs to equip the future surgical educator with the required skills to lead effective bedside rounds[2] and remains unchanged in surgical faculty. It is paramount that institutions develop educator training programs focused on developing clinical skills and teaching methods.

### Structure for Bedside Teaching Rounds

There are several ways that surgical educators can better structure bedside rounds—preround preparation, steps to take during rounds, and the postround huddle.

For preround preparation, the surgical educator should select patients with appropriate acuity and complexity based on learner level. The attending should set learning objectives and distribute teaching handout adjuncts as needed. Once the learners are assembled, the educator should discuss roles and responsibilities based on their level and orient them to the rounding plan. Educators may consider a teaching demonstration for their team.

During bedside rounds, the surgical educator can take steps to help ensure efficient, effective, and educational rounds. The first step when bringing the group into a patient's room is to set the scene—educators should introduce themselves as the physician in charge, and then introduce the students and patient to each other. In order to optimize effectiveness of teaching and minimize patient discomfort, engage the patient and utilize lay terms in the discussions carried out in front of the patient.[5]

Utilizing the subjective, objective, assessment, and plan (SOAP)-style presentation can help increase efficiency for shorter rounds.[5] The educator then prompts the students to develop a plan of care for the patient, which sets the stage for an interactive dialogue with the team. After the presentation, the educator should provide the student with balanced feedback, including a demonstration of proper physical examination technique and the opportunity for student technique correction. The surgical educator can encourage the student to enter orders discussed for the patient if the electronic medical record allows.

Once bedside rounds have concluded, a brief postround huddle provides the surgical educator with an opportunity to summarize the key learning points, promote thoughtful self-evaluation, and solicit further questions from the learners. The educator should discuss their own gaps in knowledge if present as this sets an example for the students to follow. The educator then can demonstrate to the learners how they acquire new knowledge. It sparks a willingness in the learners to identify their own deficits and gives them the skills to resolve those deficits on their own.

### One-minute Preceptor

The 1-minute preceptor model provides microskills for effective brief educational interactions by providing a structure for teaching on rounds.[8] The first step, getting a commitment, engages the learner and pushes them to synthesize data to process the clinical scenario. The educator asks the learner an open-ended patient care question, such as likely diagnosis, next steps, or etiology of disease. The second step, probing for evidence, assesses the learner's basis for the clinical assessment and challenges the individual's ability for clinical reasoning. This step establishes baseline understanding and functional knowledge. The third step is to teach a general rule or principle. This allows the educator to highlight a specific learning point and discuss pearls of wisdom pertinent to the clinical problem. The fourth step of reinforcing what was done well provides positive feedback on thought process, clinical judgment and knowledge application. The last step of correcting mistakes provides the educator the opportunity to clarify misunderstandings and encourages introspection for improvement of clinical reasoning. This 5-step process of the 1-minute preceptor model provides a reproducible educational framework to facilitate focused, efficient clinical teaching, and development of clinical reasoning.[8]

### Near-peer Teaching

One method that has been developed to address the time limitation of resident and attending physicians is the implementation of near-peer teaching. Senior medical students, typically fourth-year students with an interest in surgery or one of its subspecialties, conducts teaching rounds with junior medical students, typically third-year students on their surgery rotation. During these rounds, the junior medical students presents a patient from their service and demonstrates physical examination findings/maneuvers on the patient in front of the group of students. The senior medical student then provides feedback on the technique and presentation and leads a relevant discussion.

There are many benefits to near-peer teaching. For the senior medical student leading rounds, near-peer teaching provides them with an opportunity to take on additional responsibility and demonstrate their proficiency and knowledge and is an excellent opportunity to practice their teaching skills.[9,10] Many of the near-peer teachers report improved understanding and insight of the material that they taught because they felt they had to "learn through teaching."[10,11] The junior medical students who participated in near-peer teaching report that their rounds cover material relevant to their examinations, are an appropriate level of difficulty, resulted in improved confidence and comfort at the bedside, and report higher rates of satisfaction with the quality and amount of small-group teaching.[9-11] Additionally, both junior and senior medical students reported increased engagement, a sense of mentorship, and a comfortable and safe learning environment.[9-11] Overall, both senior and junior medical students report that near-peer teaching is an effective and positive experience.[9-12]

### Resident Versus Attending Preceptors

Resident and attending physicians play a crucial role in medical student education, although their approach in the educational process may be quite different. Attending educators focus on clinical-based problem-solving skills designed to identify areas of strengths and weaknesses in medical students' knowledge to better direct their teaching.[13] Resident educators provide students with education on day-to-day logistics and patient management topics with bedside teaching and direct supervision and instruction of clinical technical skills.[13–15] In an ideal setting, students receive instruction from both groups of educators as they play a significant role in influencing student perception of the rotation and their future career goals.[14–17] The utilization of residents as medical student educators has been found beneficial to training programs because use of resident educators is more cost-effective and time-efficient.[18]

Medical students spend a large portion of their time on their surgery rotations with the residents who may play a larger role in their education than the attending physicians.[14] Studies evaluating student perceptions of resident educators have demonstrated that surgical residents are more active in the educational process than attending educators, are easier to approach with questions, and are readily identified as mentors for the students.[14,16,17] Additionally, student perception of the surgery resident's quality of instruction has a positive, statistically significant effect on student National Board of Medical Examiners shelf examination scores.[19]

### Patient Impact from Teaching on Rounds

Some educators may feel hesitant to provide education to medical students at the patient bedside due to concerns about violating patients' privacy, imposing on the patient, or detracting from the care of the patient. In 77% to 85% of cases, pediatric and adult patients say they enjoy bedside teaching rounds, endorse an improved understanding of their disease, and perceive providers as having spent more time at the bedside.[1,20] Not only do patients report these positive impacts but also it has been demonstrated in the pediatric intensive care unit patient-parent population that residents appear more competent in the view of the family when the patient is presented at the bedside.[21] Lastly, bedside case presentations versus non-bedside case presentations do not have a difference in terms of patient outcomes.[22]

### Case Scenario: One-minute Preceptor

The resident presents a new patient with abdominal pain that came in overnight. The attending asks, "What do you think is going on?" (get a commitment). The resident says they think it is acute cholecystitis. You ask: "Ok, why do you think that?" (probe for supporting evidence). The resident describes postprandial right upper abdominal pain, leukocytosis, and an ultrasound with gallstones. You discuss other ultrasound findings that would be consistent with acute cholecystitis (teach general rules). You tell the resident that she did a good job connecting the symptoms and imaging to reach the correct diagnosis (reinforce what was done well) but should consider and rule out other similar diagnosis, such as peptic ulcer disease or symptomatic cholelithiasis (correct mistakes).

### Section Highlights/Key Takeaways

- Clinical skills in students and residents are improved through bedside teaching.
- One-minute preceptor provides a concise structure for teaching, assessing, and providing feedback on rounds.
- Near-peer teaching is an effective way to engage medical students and improves student satisfaction with benefits to both senior and junior medical students.
- Resident and attending educators provide different but complementary education to student learners.
- Teaching on rounds leads to improved patient satisfaction.

## TEACHING IN SMALL GROUPS
### Background

During the clinical years of medical school, students frequently are split into small groups, or cohorts, that rotate through core specialties and subspecialties of medicine and surgery. Students within these small groups have similar clinical and educational experiences throughout their clinical years. Small groups allow students to communicate with each other and work as a team while feeling like they are not being isolated and singled out as a learner. Although learner participation is crucial, the facilitator's ability to stimulate discussion within the small group and promote a safe learning environment has been shown to be one of the most important factors of a small group environment.[23] This section describes various types of small group practices as well as some tips for effectively facilitating small groups.

### Problem-based Learning Versus Case-based Learning

Two classic forms of small group instruction are problem-based learning (PB) and case-based learning (CBL). PBL urges learners to discover information independently, requiring students to identify gaps in their knowledge base and find supplemental resources to close these gaps.[24,25] The PBL style frequently is performed over several sessions, with learners having individual time in-between sessions to explore the various aspects of the presented problem and find answers independently rather than prepare prior to the first session.[24] Facilitators are a minor part of the typical PBL style, only available to provide expertise when learners struggle. As such, previous research has suggested that learners become better problem solvers after working through PBL-style small groups rather than lecture-only courses. This style of learning has been praised to encourage individual learning, promote learner curiosity, and stress the complexity of medicine as a field. PBL may be seen, however, as inefficient, given current time constraints of education in medical school as well as leading to flawed conclusions due to the minor role of the expert facilitator.[24]

CBL focuses on creative problem solving with an expert facilitator. A clinical case scenario is presented to learners by an expert facilitator, and the learners and facilitator work together throughout the case to reach the ultimate conclusion.[24] In this style of learning, the facilitator provides more insight and guides the discussion with topics and questions in order for learners to reach the final conclusion. Because this style of learning relies more on an expert facilitator, the CBL style has been touted as more efficient and focused than PBL. Critics of CBL believe that increased involvement of the facilitators discourages the curiosity of learners. Disbelievers of CBL also state this style of learning is more at risk of becoming a lecture by the facilitator rather than true small group learning.[24]

Although research into the 2 styles of small group learning shows mixed results,[24,26,27] the authors have found that clinical students frequently prefer the CBL style of learning. Feedback from learners has been that CBL provides more of a realistic scenario by using a clinical case to guide learning and discussion, and students also prefer to have a more guiding and active facilitator. Surgery is such a broad topic that having a facilitator guide discussion helps students stay on track and learn without finding the inevitable rabbit hole that distracts from the key point trying to be made. Srinivasan and colleagues[24] found similar attitudes of medical students at 2 different institutions, finding that both learners and facilitators preferred the guided CBL compared with PBL.

### Flipped Classroom

A more modern approach to teaching in small groups is the flipped classroom. In this style of small group, learners independently watch instructional videos and complete prework in order to encourage thought and exploration of topics prior to meeting as a group.[28–30] This allows for a more efficient and stimulating small group session, which is led by a facilitator familiar with the prework and a local expert on the topic of discussion. Surgical clerkship students overwhelmingly enjoy the flipped classroom style of instruction and the efficiency of online videos and prework.[29,30] In the authors' experience with flipped classroom–style instruction, students appreciate the modern twist on education allowing students to use multimedia and easily accessible Internet tools to discover and explore topics prior to in-depth discussion in a small group setting. A major drawback of implementing flipped classroom–style small groups into the surgical curriculum, however, is the time and monetary commitment of the facilitator to create videos, educational tools, and prework assignments prior to small group meetings. This can be managed by using established, open-access content previously created and published by national content experts. An additional limitation is the learner's commitment to completing prework activities, which must be done prior to the discussion to gain the most from the flipped classroom.

### Balancing Learner Types—Quiet versus Loud Students

In the authors' experience, for maximal effect of small group learning, the individual learners must feel comfortable and able to participate in the small group session. In order for a small group to be effective, learners must be free from fear of judgment, understand the expectations of the group, share a team identity with the group, and feel invited to participate by the facilitator.[23] Various personality and learning styles of students can potentially disrupt small group learning for other participants. It is the responsibility of the facilitator to handle these situations with care and poise.

The quiet student frequently hides within the group discussion, not speaking up when questions are asked of the group. As facilitators, the authors have found that posing initial questions to individuals and allowing the individual to answer prior to group discussion is helpful with quiet learners. It is important also to pose questions to other individuals within the group so as to not make the shy learner feel targeted. This method encourages participation by all individuals while also making sure each student has the opportunity to share in the group. Frequently, the sequestered student becomes more comfortable with sharing over time and feels more like a part of the group after this strategy is employed.

The loud student can dominate a group discussion and take away from the education for other individuals. The facilitator must recognize this type of learner early in the group discussion and should help other students participate (as discussed previously, by posing questions to other individuals). The facilitator should take care, however, to still allow the loud student to participate at the appropriate times. If the group continues to be overrun by 1 student, the facilitator may need to isolate that individual and explain the importance of group discussion.

Navigating small groups as a facilitator can be difficult; however, there are several educational groups that have published guides for educators. The Association for Medical Education in Europe has a guide for "Effective Small Group Learning" that outlines major topics for effective small group learning that is tailored to medical education.[31] This type of publication can assist with both first-time and seasoned educators.

### Case Scenario: Case-based Learning with Different Personalities

As part of the weekly conference, a patient scenario is presented to the small group of students rotating on the service. The trauma patient is hypotensive with penetrating trauma. A quiet student is asked if this patient is in shock and why and then asks the other students if they agree. The quiet student slowly starts participating more. The attending what to do next to evaluate this patient further, and the loud student who has been dominating the discussion yells that the patient needs to go to the operating room. The attending, "you may be right, but let's see what the others think." After the session, the attending pull the aggressive student aside and let him know that you want to hear his thoughts, but that the other students deserve to be heard too.

### Section Highlights/Key Takeaways

- Small groups allow students to communicate with each other and work as a team, while feeling like they are not being isolated and singled out as a learner.
- PBL urges learners to discover information independently, requiring students to identify gaps in their knowledge base and find supplemental resources to close these gaps.
- CBL focuses on creative problem solving with an expert facilitator.
- The flipped classroom utilizes prework to encourage exploration of topics prior to meeting as a group and maximize group discussion time.
- Different personalities can cause an imbalance in the group learning experience if not managed proactively.

### DISCLOSURE

The authors have no disclosures of commercial or financial conflicts.

### REFERENCES

1. Peters M, Ten Cate O. Bedside teaching in medical education: a literature review. Perspect Med Educ 2014;3(2):76–88.
2. Beigzadeh A, Bahaadinbeigy K, Adibi P, et al. Identifying the challenges to good clinical rounds: a focus-group study of medical teachers. J Adv Med Educ Prof 2019;7(2):62–73.
3. Williams KN, Ramani S, Fraser B, et al. Improving bedside teaching: findings from a focus group study of learners. Acad Med 2008;83(3):257–64.
4. Kroenke K, Omori DM, Landry FJ, et al. Bedside teaching. South Med J 1997; 90(11):1069–74.
5. Beigzadeh A, Adibi P, Bahaadinbeigy K, et al. Strategies for teaching in clinical rounds: A systematic review of the literature. J Res Med Sci 2019;24:33.
6. Katz-Sidlow RJ, Ludwig A, Miller S, et al. Smartphone use during inpatient attending rounds: prevalence, patterns and potential for distraction. J Hosp Med 2012;7(8):595–9.
7. Kim RH, Mellinger JD. Educational strategies to foster bedside teaching. Surgery 2020;167(3):532–4.
8. Gatewood E, De Gagne JC. The one-minute preceptor model: a systematic review. J Am Assoc Nurse Pract 2019;31(1):46–57.
9. Doumouras A, Rush R, Campbell A, et al. Peer-assisted bedside teaching rounds. Clin Teach 2015;12(3):197–202.
10. Lin JA, Farrow N, Lindeman BM, et al. Impact of near-peer teaching rounds on student satisfaction in the basic surgical clerkship. Am J Surg 2017;213(6): 1163–5.
11. de Menezes S, Premnath D. Near-peer education: a novel teaching program. Int J Med Educ 2016;7:160–7.
12. Wirth K, Malone B, Turner C, et al. A structured teaching curriculum for medical students improves their performance on the National Board of Medical Examiners shelf examination in surgery. Am J Surg 2015;209(4):765–70.
13. Tremonti LP, Biddle WB. Teaching behaviors of residents and faculty members. J Med Educ 1982;57(11):854–9.

14. Pelletier M, Belliveau P. Role of surgical residents in undergraduate surgical education. Can J Surg 1999;42(6):451–6.
15. Whittaker LD Jr, Estes NC, Ash J, et al. The value of resident teaching to improve student perceptions of surgery clerkships and surgical career choices. Am J Surg 2006;191(3):320–4.
16. Moore J, Parsons C, Lomas S. A resident preceptor model improves the clerkship experience on general surgery. J Surg Educ 2014;71(6):e16–8.
17. Nguyen SQ, Divino CM. Surgical residents as medical student mentors. Am J Surg 2007;193(1):90–3.
18. Kensinger CD, McMaster WG, Vella MA, et al. Residents as educators: a modern model. J Surg Educ 2015;72(5):949–56.
19. Langenfeld SJ, Helmer SD, Cusick TE, et al. Do strong resident teachers help medical students on objective examinations of knowledge? J Surg Educ 2011;68(5):350–4.
20. Gonzalo JD, Chuang CH, Huang G, et al. The return of bedside rounds: an educational intervention. J Gen Intern Med 2010;25(8):792–8.
21. Landry MA, Lafrenaye S, Roy MC, et al. A randomized, controlled trial of bedside versus conference-room case presentation in a pediatric intensive care unit. Pediatrics 2007;120(2):275–80.
22. Gamp M, Becker C, Tondorf T, et al. Effect of bedside vs. non-bedside patient case presentation during ward rounds: a systematic review and meta-analysis. J Gen Intern Med 2019;34(3):447–57.
23. Lemoine ER, Rana J, Burgin S. Teaching & learning tips 7: small-group discussion. Int J Dermatol 2018;57(5):583–6.
24. Srinivasan M, Wilkes M, Stevenson F, et al. Comparing problem-based learning with case-based learning: effects of a major curricular shift at two institutions. Acad Med 2007;82(1):74–82.
25. Wood DF. Problem based learning. BMJ 2003;326(7384):328–30.
26. Cendan JC, Silver M, Ben-David K. Changing the student clerkship from traditional lectures to small group case-based sessions benefits the student and the faculty. J Surg Educ 2011;68(2):117–20.
27. Schmidt HG, Rotgans JI, Yew EH. The process of problem-based learning: what works and why. Med Educ 2011;45(8):792–806.
28. Lewis CE, Chen DC, Relan A. Implementation of a flipped classroom approach to promote active learning in the third-year surgery clerkship. Am J Surg 2018;215(2):298–303.
29. Liebert CA, Lin DT, Mazer LM, et al. Effectiveness of the surgery core clerkship flipped classroom: a prospective cohort trial. Am J Surg 2016;211(2):451–7.e451.
30. Liebert CA, Mazer L, Bereknyei Merrell S, et al. Student perceptions of a simulation-based flipped classroom for the surgery clerkship: a mixed-methods study. Surgery 2016;160(3):591–8.
31. Edmunds S, Brown G. Effective small group learning: AMEE Guide No. 48. Med Teach 2010;32(9):715–26.

# Effective Large Group Teaching for General Surgery

Samantha L. Tarras, MD, Jock Thacker, MD,
David L. Bouwman, MD, David A. Edelman, MD, MSHPEd*

## KEYWORDS

- Large group teaching • Surgical education • Effective lecture
- Synchronous learning • Asynchronous learning • Hybrid learning

## KEY POINTS

- Students need to participate actively to become learners.
- Converting from classic passive lecturing to a modern format using active learning will increase lecture effectiveness.
- It is imperative for surgeons charged with surgical education in general, and specifically lecturing, to adopt modern methods and to improve their skill in the use of established modern practices.
- This practice will increase the effectiveness of their efforts and meet the expectations of students already familiar with modern methods.

## INTRODUCTION

Large group settings, such as grand rounds, clerkship lectures, and core basic science lectures, display no signs of disappearing; most surgeons charged with this education have received no formal training.[1,2] The lecture remains the most common method of educating large groups.[3] Although the factors required for an excellent lecture are known, their inconsistent application results in wide variation of effectiveness and leaves much room for improvement. Long-standing principles of rhetoric and more recent advances in neuroscience, cognitive science, learning models, and teaching theory each play a role in achieving effectiveness.[4] This article makes recommendations for creating and delivering lectures including active learning opportunities. The discussion includes modern innovations in information technology (IT) that support teaching methods beyond the lecture for large groups. Effective lecturing skill cannot be gained by reading this article, because skills are only acquired by persistent

The Michael and Marian Ilitch Department of Surgery, Wayne State University School of Medicine, Suite 400, 3990 John R, Detroit, MI 48201, USA
* Corresponding author.
*E-mail address:* dedelman@med.wayne.edu

Surg Clin N Am 101 (2021) 565–576
https://doi.org/10.1016/j.suc.2021.05.004
0039-6109/21/© 2021 Elsevier Inc. All rights reserved.
surgical.theclinics.com

deliberate practice.[5] This article outlines a clear goal and provides selected references to sources for additional study.

Lectures began at medieval universities as direct readings of scarce texts to audiences otherwise without access. The modern lecture rests on the same premise of an expert transmitting knowledge to a passive audience. However, passive transmission misses the opportunity to promote active initiative by learners to build their own meaning. Active learning methods consistently report improved educational outcomes in many settings in higher education.[1,6,7]

The obsolete lecture persists for several reasons.[8] Lectures with their large audiences are perceived by course administrators to effectively deliver information.[3] Commissioning a lecture documents educational effort; often, a lecture is the only locally available option. Lecturing is well-accepted and carries a long history[9]; lecturers grew up with lectures and the majority of today's students still expect these familiar sessions. Lectures can stimulate interest, explain concepts, provide structure for new information, and direct student learning.[10] The lecture carries the potency of a live performance event.[11] Notes that capture this structure are valuable study guides for new material.

Lectures have negative characteristics related to their failure to promote active learning. Passive information transfer leaves little opportunity to process, connect, or critically appraise the new knowledge offered. The cognitive load of encoding and recording the narrative stream in notes may exceed the learners' capacity, resulting in poor engagement, lower commitment to courses, low motivation, poor participation, and social isolation.[12] Problems increase and change as class size increases: anonymity, disempowerment, lack of engagement, failure to resolve misunderstandings, and loss of feedback.[13] Some students respond by engaging in poor behaviors including arriving late, leaving early, or even skipping all together.[14] Lecturing is also ill-suited to teaching skills and has difficulty in modifying attitudes or developing higher order thinking.[15]

The negative aspects of the passive transmission model can be decreased by introducing opportunities for active learning.[6] Active learning theory was articulated more than 30 years ago as a learner-centric method where the learner is strongly engaged in actively acquiring knowledge and building meaning by participation, social reinforcement, integration of new knowledge with existing knowledge, and practicing synthesis and judgment.[16] Active learning is associated with better educational results for learners, including increased levels of content acquisition and retention, and the development of higher order cognition, such as critical thinking, evaluation, and synthesis.[17,18] Active learning principles align with modern adult learning theory,[19] experiential learning theory,[20–22] and older more classic approaches like Vygotsky's "zone of proximal development" or Gagne's conditions of learning.[23,24] Classroom teaching using active learning methods provides resources for planned activities leading to autocorrecting collaborations with only suggestions and error correction by facilitators.

Focused, efficient lectures have time to include active learning opportunities. Additional participation occurs because students with mature learning skills (self-awareness, self-assessment, self-regulation, and goal setting) can convert lecture content that is outwardly passive into active learning. This phenomenon requires the passive lecture format to be crafted and delivered as a compelling presentation aligned with the needs and goals of the audience. A lecture managing time and technology to insert active learning opportunities requires effort comparable with the production of a live theater performance in terms of the preparation and rehearsal involved.

## HOW TO CREATE AN EFFECTIVE LECTURE

The steps presented in this article organize the requirements for creating and delivering an effective lecture with active learning content. Two types of entries arise: those associated with adherence to long-standing principles of rhetoric and those introducing active learning methods.

### Step 1. Get the Important Details at the Time the Lecture Is Proposed

A lecture is not usually given on the initiative of the surgical lecturer. Typically, a departmental authority, a course director, or the residency training program director requests or assigns the lecturer with a topic. There are details necessary for preparing an effective lecture. Keep them in mind using the maxim: when, where, what, why, and to whom.

"When" concerns the date for the lecture and the amount of time allotted. After checking availability, insist on adequate lead time before accepting the assignment. Preparing a new lecture, even on familiar material, involves many hours that might require weeks of lead time depending on other workload. The 1-hour length of typical surgical lectures is nominal; the presentation should fit comfortably into 45 minutes.

"Where" determines available infrastructure (AV set-up, computer availability, and applications available such as audience polling, availability of online connection, and cellphone reception). The site sets the level of connection with the audience.

"What," "why," and "to whom" are inter-related factors conditioning the educational objectives for the lecture. "What" sets the topic, but adequate focus requires considering the specific purpose (why) and audience specifics (to whom). Whatever the topic, engaging the audience effectively requires knowing their existing level of knowledge, their level of learning skills, and their goals. Surgeons and residents expect objectives at the apex levels of Bloom's triangular taxonomy of knowledge (create, evaluate, and analyze) and benefit from the concise activation of the required knowledge base for the topic.[25,26] Meanwhile students need structure to organize facts into concepts supporting higher order thinking. The short-term goals of learners focus on impending assessments (course final examinations, US Medical Licensing Examinations, American Board of Surgery Inservice Training Examinations, or American Board of Surgery certification and maintenance requirements). Determine whether the audience is registered in a learning management system (LMS; such as Blackboard Learn, Canvas, or Moodle) that facilitates online access to preread materials and course handouts before the lecture. A 1-hour lecture can address 4 to 6 well-articulated learning objectives if they matched to audience level and focused.

### Step 2. Choose the Objectives to Be Presented

The surgical lecturer will need to create or adjust the list of objectives depending on how well step 1 was executed. Rewrite objectives as necessary to focus and align them with the needs and expectations of the audience. Decrease the number of objectives if there are too many by combining related topics and demoting objectives for which excellent outside sources exist (refer learners to a handout). Add objectives if needed that fill logical holes in the presentation.

The lecture must fit these objectives into a presentation, structuring facts and concepts logically to promote engagement, comprehension, effective encoding, analysis, and application. Most objectives should be in Bloom's cognitive knowledge domain, because lectures are inefficient for achieving educational goals in the affective or psychomotor domains.

### Step 3. Organize the Objectives Logically and Configure the Presentation on a Modular Basis

The main problem for the lecturer is fitting a presentation into the time allotted while including opportunities for active learning. This process requires ruthless reduction of passive portions of the presentation to avoid including only token amounts of active learning. One approach is "chunking," as applied by authors of online education-based on modular videos.[27,28] This top-down method begins with the objectives and lists only the concepts and facts essential for achieving each objective. Lecture effectiveness is boosted by providing an opportunity for active learning within each module. Additional material is used sparingly to support advancement of arguments that organize the module into a coherent entity. Usually this construct suggests the design for 1 or 2 presentation slides. The treatment of each objective begins with an introduction linking it to the prior portion of the presentation. This part is followed by a short exposition of content and an active learning element. The module concludes with a summary reinforcing the content, clearly denoting the critical take aways, and signaling transition to the next segment.

Many tactics promoting active learning can be accommodated within a lecture.[29] A poll by hand raising at a decision point allows correction of misunderstandings (consumes 1–2 minutes). The solicitation of open questions is more time consuming, but yields important feedback to the presenter on audience engagement and comprehension (allow several minutes per question). Audience polling by digital applications using clickers or cellphones can present multiple choice questions with tabulation and display of results (consumes 1–2 minutes per question); well-designed distracting choices can trigger a discussion of difficulties with the presentation. Buzz groups (2 or 3 adjacent audience member huddling) collaborate on a consensus answer to a question with an aggregate report to entire audience (set up, discussion, and reporting will take 6–8 minutes). Thinking out loud by the speaker while solving an example task demonstrates use of newly integrated knowledge. That portion of the presentation will proceed at half speed. The presenter can also appeal directly to the audience for reflection and the formation of an opinion (1–2 minutes).

This top-down minimalist construction (using IT resources) frees up the time required by insertion of the active learning opportunity. The completion of each segment punctuates the presentation, avoiding the documented loss of attention occurring during passive lectures. These breakpoints allow a reprise that can rescue confused learners who have disengaged from the lecture. Active learning opportunities consume extra time when initially used by inexperienced speakers and audiences not expecting these techniques.

Visual media can add significant value to a presentation, following a few rules to ensure effectiveness. An audience member reading the slide should find an organized succinct representation in image or text that parallels and augments the speaker's message. Duplication of the speaker's narrative is wasteful and completely dissociated content is destructive of audience engagement. The standard recommendations for designing slides are available online.[30,31] Use a template with 40-point headings and 28-point text, limit text content to a terse outline form with 3 to 6 bullets per slide, and only use images that clearly reinforce the narrative. Use videos rarely; they consume time and interrupt the flow of the presentation. If used, videos must be edited down to pertinent content and seamless integration into the presentation software is required.

### Step 4. Create a Narrative Script

Humans avidly listen to well-told stories. Lecturers should tell compelling stories using the principles of creative writing. Begin by engaging the audience's attention, activate prior knowledge, and connect content to what they already know. List the objectives to be accomplished and the skills they promote. Provide a map of the lecture's structure and promise to identify and emphasize crucial concepts for take away. Provide advice on using slide handouts as a skeleton for notes. Invite the audience to listen and watch the speaker rather than reading the slides and taking notes. Emphasize the development of meta-cognitive skills (self-assessment, self-regulation, time management, and effective study group participation).[32]

Proceed through each module with a brief introduction followed by core concepts of the objective presented coherently and with enthusiasm. This advice stands in contrast with the unemotional formal style of a scientific report. Delay introducing caveats and counterexamples that might sow confusion until after the basic positive structure is established. Avoid digression, including only the elements identified in step 3 that clearly contribute to the logical structure of the presentation. Include advanced ideas of interest to only a few audience members by reference to your handouts. Remedial elements required by other audience members are also referred to the reading list. The goal is to address the level of discussion to the average audience member as identified from step 1. Use active learning breaks as a time of respite for review and reflection that reinforce critical concepts. Resist showing off arcane trivia. Restrict the expository portion of the lecture into the least time required within each module. Take care to avoid gaps in reasoning or inclusion of logical inconsistencies, because these elements may derail learners; use simple declarative propositions. Thoroughly link new knowledge structures to known material. Conclude each segment with a summary reprise that identifies core concepts. Authoring this narrative is a crucial basis for further preparation.

### Step 5. Time the Narrative and Coordinate the Visual Media

Read the narrative script out loud and mark the slide changes. Do not speed read; 100 words per minute is a target for avoiding cognitive overload; dense material requires a slower rate. Remember to pause the appropriate length of time for the insertion of active learning episodes and allow time to address the feedback from those activities. Answering questions carries high value if the audience requires reengagement. Defer distracting questions until after the lecture, while concentrating on questions from learners with problems of understanding. If a confused audience cannot ask a good question, the lecturer can pose a frequently asked question from a previous instance of the lecture. When there are too many good questions for the allotted time, offer to accommodate them after the presentation.

Recording the reading allows review and deferment of timing, which must otherwise be noted manually during the reading. Ideally, the script will be narrated in 40 to 45 minutes. Shorten by editing that restructures awkward sections or deletes whole nonessential passages. Seek to refer additional content to the preread material. Resist solving time over-runs by decreasing the active learning component of the lecture. If the initial read through is the right duration, still edit it down using the same rules to make room for additional active learning. Remember to alter slides to stay in agreement with the presentation and to cue slide changes at appropriate times.

### Step 6. Choreograph the Delivery

Using the edited script and media, practice the delivery of the presentation. Use gestures and address the slides; use pauses for critical statements. If available, use an observer or video tape for timing and critique. The goal is to mark awkward sections for later revision and to cue in slide changes and effective gestures. Note whether the tempo for each segment between slide changes was appropriate and adjust it. Often the total time required will be too long for the intended presentation. This step provides a last chance to adjust the presentation structurally. Find alternatives for difficult or overtime sections that smooth or shorten the presentation. If no alternative is available, consider deletion of an entire noncore objective from the presentation. There are always solutions if the author has allowed enough time for preparation. These repetitive run-throughs allow speakers to abandon their scripts and create abbreviated notes for delivery. If a script is used at presentation, do not read from it.

This reworking polishes the presentation and frees up the presenter to project personality, affect, and enthusiasm during the lecture. Audiences observe speaker affect closely seeking role models and registering the attitudes displayed. This stage presence can offer opportunity to teach objectives in the affective domain. Truly effective lectures require repeated rehearsal.

### Step 7. Giving the Lecture

By the lecture date, the preparation should be long finished. Arrive early to interface with the AV aide in setting up your computer or loading your presentation. Adjust the microphone, sound check the audio volumes, and test the slide controller. It is important to start on time with a presentation designed to fill the time allotted. Audiences expect on time release and even a 5-minute late start will rush a presentation. Have a back-up plan for shortening the presentation in the event of a major interruption like equipment failure. Trust your preparations and fall into the rhythms of your practice session, but run a timer on the podium to ensure that your planned tempo is maintained. Remember that the adrenergic priming accompanying performance anxiety can speed up delivery to a dysfunctional level. The best solution for stage fright is compulsive preparation and practice sessions that build confidence.

Effective lectures are performances. They tarry dramatically over important points and use varied dynamics for effect; they inject enthusiasm, wonder, or even disappointment as appropriate.

## ADDITIONAL FACTORS THAT IMPROVE THE EFFECTIVENESS OF LECTURES
### Lecturer-Based General Factors

Lecturing is a skill improved by deliberate practice accumulated over time. Making the conscious effort to improve at every opportunity increases the effectiveness of future lectures and decreases the effort required to produce them. This deliberate practice depends on feedback. After each event, lecturers should review their performances noting what went well and what caused difficulty. Seek out audience survey results; all lectures approved for continuing medical education credit are surveyed, as are most medical student attended lectures.

Surgeons have access to educational programs of the American College of Surgeons that are designed to improve educator skills; these offerings range from sessions during the annual American College of Surgeons meetings to a weeklong retreat entitled "Surgeons as Educators."[33] Many medical schools and local educational consortia sponsor development workshops for local educators. Extensive published or online self-improvement materials are also available.

### Organization-Based General Factors

The organization assigning the lecture, and frequently the employer of the lecturer, has the primary responsibility to determine the objectives of the lecture and to align these educational goals with planned assessment methods. The most objective measure of effectiveness is based on valid assessments of learning outcomes. Lectures gain effectiveness when alignment is accurate and when lecturers are given well-defined objectives.

The organization is responsible for the services that support lecture presentations. At a minimum, this responsibility includes the audiovisual setup in the auditorium, but it may include the capacity for live streaming or digital recording. Large educational institutions usually subscribe to an LMS, as mentioned in step 1. In addition to prelecture preparations, these systems can be used to collect feedback or provide online access to the lecture synchronously and/or asynchronously for registered attendees or a wider audience.

The organization may sponsor faculty development courses in house or send educators to the American College of Surgeons educator courses. The overall effectiveness of an educational effort is improved by a commitment to faculty development as educators. Educational organizations can increase the effectiveness by extended efforts to develop metacognitive maturity in their learners as addressed elsewhere in this article.

### Student-Based General Factors

Lectures are effective when learners arrive rested, motivated, and prepared to learn. Students possess some level of learning skill as a result of long-term development. Learning a skill is a specific application of meta-cognition (literally thinking about thinking), which is based on high-level knowledge about cognitive processes. Students with mature meta-cognition manage their roles as learners to achieve better outcomes in educational programs and to become accomplished self-directed learners. Lectures become more effective as the aggregate meta-cognitive level of the audience increases.

## NONTRADITIONAL LARGE GROUP EDUCATION

Nontraditional large group education depends on using educational applications on digital platforms. An LMS is absolutely required for moving beyond lectures to flipped classroom techniques or other blended learning methods.[34–36] Full-featured LMSs may contain authoring software for generating new content for online learning, but freestanding authoring applications are also available. Electronic learning opens up greater access, higher efficacy of educational effort, cost effectiveness, learner flexibility, and interactivity.[37] Widespread high-speed Internet availability combined with advances in personal digital devices has resulted in an accelerated development of educational applications. One way to overview this range of available functionality is to classify these methods as synchronous, asynchronous, or hybrid.

### Synchronous Learning

Synchronous learning happens in real time where students, classmates, and the instructor gather to interact in a specific virtual place through an online medium and time. Examples include video conferencing, teleconferencing, live chatting, and live stream lectures. The advantages of synchronous learning include classroom engagement, dynamic learning, and instructional depth. Synchronous learning allows for active discussion, immediate feedback, personal engagement, and interaction with instructors. No significant difference has been reported in national licensing examination performance between medical students receiving their lectures through synchronous videoconferencing as opposed to those attending live lectures.[38] Medical students prefer to exploit a variety of online methods: podcasts, webinars, narrated presentations, synchronous small group tutorials, and asynchronous formative assessments combined with later synchronous large group feedback.[39]

The disadvantages of synchronous learning include the requirement for prescheduling and technical difficulties in getting participants fully connected. A recent report reviewing the use of videoconferencing tools for anatomy teaching found restrictions surrounding the Human Tissue Act, with limited online accessibility in comparison with real-time sessions.[40] The effective use of online educational content requires reliable access for students and educators. Connectivity was reported to be the most important factor in the use of videoconferencing platforms.[41] Incidents of malicious hacking intended to disrupt teaching sessions have been reported.[42] As online learning becomes a predominant modality, institutional policy must mandate standard security practices: secure links, limits on link forwarding, password protection, secure participant registration, the ability to mute participants, control of chatrooms, and restricting the right to annotate and to screen share. Students with limited resources require support for broadband access. Support is also required for faculty seeking to incorporate technology into their teaching.

### Asynchronous Learning

Asynchronous learning depends only on the learner's schedule. The reading assignments, recorded lectures to be viewed, tasks to be completed, and assessment examinations are available online at any time, although completion deadlines may be set. No scheduled virtual meetings occur. Methods of asynchronous online learning include self-guided lesson modules, individual tutoring programs, video episodes, virtual libraries, posted lecture notes, and exchanges across discussion boards or social media. The advantages of asynchronous learning include flexible goal setting, the ability to self-pace, and affordability. Disadvantages include the risk of isolation, the risk of apathy, and dependence on the presence of basic meta-cognition. Some learners require clearly enforced expectations, immediate feedback, and social interaction, which are difficult to deliver in an asynchronous learning environment.

### Hybrid Learning

Hybrid learning, or blended learning, is the combination of traditional in-person learning with varying amounts of either asynchronous or synchronous learning.[43] Blended learning represents a promising approach for health education by combining the advantage of traditional learning with e-learning.[44] It is now used widely in education.[45] A systematic review of blended learning in medical education identifies a potential to improve clinical competencies among health students.[46] Blended learning displays consistent positive effects in comparison with no intervention and is as effective as nonblended instruction for knowledge acquisition in the health professions.[47] Surgical residents exposed to blended learning reported high satisfaction from working through modular, locally produced, audiovisual curriculum and participating in hands-on sessions simulating operations. The cost of these programs was affordable and allowed use trainees with work-hour limits.[48] Video-based coaching outperforms laparoscopic skills training in improving performance.[49]

### Team-Based Learning

Team-based learning for large group instruction divides the group into multiple teams of 5 to 7 members who collaborate in solving tasks and synthesizing answers. The groups are overseen by 1 faculty mediator and the method emphasizes knowledge construction and application by the learners as an alternative to passive knowledge transmission.[50] Preassigned work is completed before the session. Readiness assessment tests are given to individuals and then to the team for consensus answers. Each team then solves "real-life" problem using concepts from the discussions of pre-work and defends their management decisions in intergroup discussion.[50–52] Team-based learning has been adopted in most medical school curricula.[53] Team-based learning is documented to increase learners' leadership, communication, and team-work skills.[54] Faculty require team-based learning training before the development of a course. Faculty attitudes toward team-based learning are positive. Team-based learning increases course preparation work and student engagement.[55] Team-based learning in surgery clerkships is described as positive; medical students benefit from team-based learning with no loss of fundamental surgery knowledge.[56]

## SUMMARY

Students need to participate actively to become learners. Converting from classic passive lecturing to a modern format using active learning will increase lecture effectiveness. Modern IT infrastructure can enable this change but the isolated surgical lecturer devoid of IT support can still optimize lectures by injecting active learning. Modern IT is not a panacea, but investing effort in learning to apply it will increase the effectiveness of lectures. It is imperative for surgeons charged with surgical education in general, and specifically lecturing, to adopt modern methods and to improve their skill in the use of established modern practices. This process will increase the effectiveness of their efforts and meet the expectations of students already familiar with modern methods.

## ACKNOWLEDGMENT

Received funding support from The Fund of Surgical Education and Education Research a program of the Detroit International Research and Education Foundation.

## REFERENCES

1. Sweeney WB. Teaching surgery to medical students. Clin Colon Rectal Surg 2012;25(3):127–33.
2. Dickinson KJ, Bass BL, Pei KY. The Current Evidence for Defining and Assessing Effectiveness of Surgical Educators: A Systematic Review. World J Surg 2020;44(10):3214-23.
3. Schmidt HG, Wagener SL, Smeets GACM, et al. On the use and misuse of lectures in higher education. Health Professions Education 2015;1(1):12–8.
4. Council NR. How people learn: brain, mind, experience, and school. Expanded Edition. Washington, DC: The National Academies Press; 2000. p. 384.
5. Ericsson KA, Harwell KW. Deliberate practice and proposed limits on the effects of practice on the acquisition of expert performance: why the original definition matters and recommendations for future research. Front Psychol 2019; 10(2396):2396.
6. Michael J. Where's the evidence that active learning works? Adv Physiol Educ 2006;30(4):159–67.
7. Cloonan M, Fingeret AL. Developing teaching materials for learners in surgery. Surgery 2020;167(4):689–92.
8. French S, Kennedy G. Reassessing the value of university lectures. Teach Higher Educ 2017;22(6):639–54.

9. Geske J. Overcoming the drawbacks of the large lecture class. Coll Teach 1992; 40(4):151–4.

10. Mulryan-Kyne C. Teaching large classes at college and university level: challenges and opportunities. Teach Higher Education 2010;15(2):175–85.

11. Wongtrakul W, Dangprapai Y. Effects of Live Lecture Attendance on the Academic Achievement of Preclinical Medical Students. Med Sci Educator 2020;1523–30.

12. Gibbs, Graham, Alan Jenkins, and Jenkins Alan, eds. *Teaching large classes in higher education: How to maintain quality with reduced resources.* Psychology Press, 1992.

13. Biggs J, Tang C. Teaching for quality learning at university. Buckingham: SRHE and Open University Press. Biggs, J.(2014). Constructive alignment in university teaching. HERDSA Rev Higher Education 1999;1:5–22.

14. Carbone E. Students behaving badly in large classes. New Dir Teach Learn 1999; 1999(77):35–43.

15. McKimm J, Jollie C, Cantillon P. ABC of learning and teaching: web based learning. BMJ 2003;326(7394):870–3.

16. Michael, Joel, and Modell, Harold I.. Active Learning in Secondary and College Science Classrooms: A Working Model for Helping the Learner To Learn. N.p., Taylor & Francis, 2003.

17. Terenzini PT, Springer L, Pascarella ET, et al. Influences affecting the development of students' critical thinking skills. Res High Educ 1995;36(1):23–39.

18. Weaver RR, Qi J. Classroom organization and participation: college students' perceptions. J Higher Educ 2005;76(5):570–601.

19. Knowles, M. S. "The modern practice of adult education (revised edition)." *New York: Cambridge Book Company* (1980).

20. Engels PT, de Gara C. Learning styles of medical students, general surgery residents, and general surgeons: implications for surgical education. BMC Med Educ 2010;10(1):51.

21. Kolb DA. Experience as the source of learning and development. *Upper Sadle River: Prentice Hall* (1984).

22. Kolb AY, Kolb DA. Learning styles and learning spaces: enhancing experiential learning in higher education. Amle 2005;4(2):193–212.

23. Vygotsky LS. Mind in Society: The Development of Higher Psychological Processes. United Kingdom: Harvard University Press; 1980.

24. Gagne RM. Instruction and the conditions of learning. Psychol Sch Learn Views Learner 1974;1:153–75.

25. Crookston KP, Richter DM. Teaching and learning apheresis medicine: the Bermuda Triangle in education. J Clin Apher 2010;25(6):338–46.

26. Bloom BS. Taxonomy of educational objectives. Vol. 1: cognitive domain, vol. 20. New York: McKay; 1956. p. 24.

27. Ruiz JG, Mintzer MJ, Issenberg SB. Learning objects in medical education. Med Teach 2006;28(7):599–605.

28. The Cambridge handbook of Multimedia learning. 2 ed. Cambridge Handbooks in Psychology. Cambridge: Cambridge University Press; 2014.

29. Cantillon P. Teaching large groups. BMJ 2003;326(7386):437.

30. Mahajan R, Gupta K, Gupta P, et al. Multimedia instructional design principles: moving from theoretical rationale to practical applications. Indian Pediatr 2020; 57(6):555–60.

31. Churchill D. Conceptual model learning objects and design recommendations for small screens. J Educ Technology Soc 2011;14(1):203–16.

32. Medina MS, Castleberry AN, Persky AM. Strategies for improving learner meta-cognition in health professional education. Am J Pharm Educ 2017;81(4):78.
33. DaRosa DA, Folse JR, Reznick RK, et al. Description and evaluation of the Surgeons as Educators course. J Am Coll Surg 1996;183(5):499–505.
34. Chick RC, Clifton GT, Peace KM, et al. Using technology to maintain the education of residents during the COVID-19 pandemic. J Surg Education 2020;77(4): 729–32.
35. Ramnanan CJ, Pound LD. Advances in medical education and practice: student perceptions of the flipped classroom. Adv Med Educ Pract 2017;8:63–73.
36. Lewis CE, Chen DC, Relan A. Implementation of a flipped classroom approach to promote active learning in the third-year surgery clerkship. Am J Surg 2018; 215(2):298–303.
37.. Ehlers, Ulf-Daniel, and Pawlowski, Jan Martin. Handbook on Quality and Standardisation in E-Learning. Germany, Physica-Verlag, 2006.
38. Hortos K, Sefcik D, Wilson SG, et al. Synchronous videoconferencing: impact on achievement of medical students. Teach Learn Med 2013;25(3):211–5.
39. Joseph JP, Joseph AO, Conn G, et al. COVID-19 pandemic—medical education adaptations: the power of students, staff and technology. Med Sci Educ 2020;1–2. https://doi.org/10.1007/s40670-020-01038-4.
40. Allsop S, Hollifield M, Huppler L, et al. Using videoconferencing to deliver anatomy teaching to medical students on clinical placements. Transl Res Anat 2020; 19:100059.
41. Sidpra J, Gaier C, Reddy N, et al. Sustaining education in the age of COVID-19: a survey of synchronous web-based platforms. Quant Imaging Med Surg 2020; 10(7):1422–7.
42. Jane W. "Coronavirus: Racist "zoombombing" at virtual synagogue." BBC News 2020.
43. Bonk, Curtis J., and Graham, Charles R. The Handbook of Blended Learning: Global Perspectives, Local Designs. Germany, Wiley, 2012.
44. Makhdoom N, Khoshhal KI, Algaidi S, et al. 'Blended learning' as an effective teaching and learning strategy in clinical medicine: a comparative cross-sectional university-based study. J taibah Univ Med Sci 2013;8(1):12–7.
45. Norberg A, Dziuban CD, Moskal PD. A time-based blended learning model. On the Horizon; Vol 19, No 3, pp. 207-16.
46. Rowe M, Frantz J, Bozalek V. The role of blended learning in the clinical education of healthcare students: a systematic review. Med Teach 2012;34(4):e216–21.
47. Liu Q, Peng W, Zhang F, et al. The effectiveness of blended learning in health professions: systematic review and meta-analysis. J Med Internet Res 2016; 18(1):e2.
48. AlJamal YN, Ali SM, Ruparel RK, et al. The rationale for combining an online audiovisual curriculum with simulation to better educate general surgery trainees. Surgery 2014;156(3):723–8.
49. Singh P, Aggarwal R, Tahir M, et al. A randomized controlled study to evaluate the role of video-based coaching in training laparoscopic skills. Ann Surg 2015; 261(5):862–9.
50. Parmelee D, Michaelsen LK, Cook S, et al. Team-based learning: a practical guide: AMEE guide no. 65. Med Teach 2012;34(5):e275–87.
51. Kibble JD, Bellew C, Asmar A, et al. Team-based learning in large enrollment classes. Adv Physiol Educ 2016;40(4):435–42.
52. Johnson C. Team-based learning for health professions education: a guide to using small groups for improving learning. J Chiropractic Educ 2009;23(1):47–8.

53. Haidet P, Kubitz K, McCormack WT. Analysis of the team-based learning literature: TBL comes of age. J Excell Coll Teach 2014;25(3–4):303–33.

54. Haidet P, Levine RE, Parmelee DX, et al. Perspective: guidelines for reporting team-based learning activities in the medical and health sciences education literature. Acad Med 2012;87(3):292–9.

55. Reimschisel T, Herring AL, Huang J, et al. A systematic review of the published literature on team-based learning in health professions education. Med Teach 2017;39(12):1227–37.

56. Kaminski AD, Babbitt KM, McCarthy MC, et al. Team-based learning in the surgery clerkship: impact on student examination scores, evaluations, and perceptions. J Surg Educ 2019;76(2):408–13.

# Teaching and Evaluating Nontechnical Skills for General Surgery

Ryland Stucke, MD[a], Kari M. Rosenkranz, MD[b],*

## KEYWORDS

- Nontechnical skills • Intraoperative leadership • Situational awareness • Teamwork
- Communication • Decision making

## KEY POINTS

- Nontechnical skills are critical to enhancing surgical team dynamics and ensuring the best possible patient outcomes.
- Nontechnical skills encompass several domains, including leadership, situational awareness, decision making, communication, and teamwork.
- Nontechnical skills are difficult to teach, measure, and evaluate but should be an integral part of assessment for surgical trainees and staff surgeons.

## INTRODUCTION

The importance of technical skills in surgery has long been understood. Surgeons require manual dexterity, hand-eye coordination, and psychomotor skills in order to safely complete an operation. However, clinical outcomes in current surgical practice depend on many factors beyond the surgeon's technical prowess. Nontechnical skills in the operating room are now recognized as an important skill set for successful surgeons in minimizing adverse events and enhancing the work environment.[1,2] Nontechnical skills are the cognitive and social skills by which surgeons make and execute decisions in the perioperative environment. The nontechnical skills critical to surgical excellence include leadership, communication and teamwork, situation awareness, and decision making. Lapses in these abilities are responsible for a large proportion of medical errors.[3,4] These skills are not innate, but are teachable and can be evaluated and refined over time.[2] The common aims of nontechnical skills training are to

[a] Fellow in Advanced GI and Minimally Invasive Surgery, Department of Surgery, Oregon Health and Sciences University, 3181 S.W. Sam Jackson Park Road, Portland, Oregon 97239, USA; [b] Associate Professor of Surgery, Department of Surgery, Geisel School of Medicine, Dartmouth-Hitchcock Medical Center, 1 Medical Center Drive, Lebanon, New Hampshire 03756, USA
* Corresponding author.
*E-mail address:* kari.m.rosenkranz@hitchcock.org

Surg Clin N Am 101 (2021) 577–586
https://doi.org/10.1016/j.suc.2021.05.005
0039-6109/21/© 2021 Elsevier Inc. All rights reserved.

improve patient safety and maximize surgical outcomes for patients. With improvements in nontechnical skills, respect for team members is also heightened and the work environment improves.[5] This improvement can lead to decreased provider burnout, which also leads to improved patient outcomes, increased career longevity, and heightened engagement of the surgical workforce. This article reviews existing frameworks for defining nontechnical skills, educational models to train these skills, and assessment tools. It then provides evidence-based recommendations for surgical training programs, hospitals, and health systems to incorporate nontechnical skills training and evaluation. All surgeons, regardless of experience or seniority, must be held accountable for their nontechnical skills in order ensure the highest possible quality outcomes.

## HISTORICAL PERSPECTIVE

Surgical volume is increasing annually in all economic environments, with an estimated 312.9 million operations performed in 2012, a 33.6% increase from just 8 years prior.[6] In addition, medical knowledge is estimated to double every 73 days.[7] In order to safely perform the increasing volume of surgery in an era of rapidly expanding medical knowledge, the paradigm for the delivery of safe surgical care has evolved. Modern surgery is now defined by dynamic technology, team-based care, and a systematic approach to quality and safety.[8] Simultaneous with the increase in surgical knowledge and volume, institutions have increased awareness of patient safety and harm reduction. This movement was initially catalyzed by the United States Institution of Medicine Report, *To Err is Human*, published in 1999,[9] and the United Kingdom Department of Health report, *An Organization with a Memory*, published in 2000.[10] The World Health Organization (WHO) surgical safety checklist was introduced in 2008 as an effort to address intraoperative safety.[11] Implementation of the WHO surgical checklist is an acknowledgment of the just culture of the operating room, an environment in which every team member has a voice, and a tangible example of the importance of nontechnical skills in improving the care of surgical patients.[12]

Technical skills are necessary for safe surgery, but there is a growing body of evidence that technical skills alone are not sufficient to provide high-quality surgical care and ensure patient safety. Significant research from the past 2 decades has identified that nontechnical factors are key contributors to adverse patient outcomes and near misses in the perioperative environment.[3,13–19] In 1 study of surgical patients experiencing complications, 66% of errors occurred during the intraoperative phase of care. Systems errors, rather than isolated technical mistakes, contributed to the adverse outcome in 86% of cases.[3] The 2010 Scottish Audit of Surgical Mortality reported that only 4.3% of adverse operative events were related to technical errors, although most complications resulted from poor decision making.[18] In 2014, surgical error led to 7 million complications and 1 million deaths globally; most of these outcomes were attributable to nontechnical errors.[19] The ability to think critically, problem solve, lead a team, and communicate effectively is vitally important to patient safety and high-quality care. The perioperative environment has moved beyond the historical surgeon-centric paradigm to a team-based, multidisciplinary care model that focuses on broader metrics of success, including quality, safety, and patient satisfaction.[13,14,20]

## DEFINITIONS AND KEY TERMS

In 2006, a group at the University of Aberdeen in Scotland performed a comprehensive literature review in order to ascertain the nontechnical skills that are most critical for surgeons to possess in order to ensure the best patient outcomes. Based on this work, a formal framework for both teaching and assessing nontechnical skills for surgeons (NOTSS) was systematically developed.[21–25] Before these efforts, no validated framework existed for teaching or assessing nontechnical skills in the operating room. Conceptual frameworks were, in part, adapted from other high-risk industries, including aviation and nuclear power, which had previously emphasized nontechnical skills to improve safety and performance.[21,26] In the NOTSS paradigm, nontechnical skills are grouped into 4 major categories: (1) decision-making skills, (2) leadership skills, (3) communication skills, and (4) situational awareness. Each category is further described by 3 elements that exemplify surgical behaviors. Taken together, this framework provides a shared vocabulary and a mental model for understanding and teaching nontechnical skills for surgeons.[22–25]

Nontechnical skills have been alternatively represented by 3 personal skill domains: interpersonal skills (communication and teamwork), cognitive skills (decision making and situational awareness), and personal resources (ability to cope with stress and fatigue).[27] However, the component behaviors of this alternate framework overlap without exception.

### Situation Awareness

Situation awareness is the recognition of what is going on around oneself, a perception of how others are reacting in the situation, and a recognition of changes in the situation. Situation awareness encompasses the ability to perceive the context of the task being performed, including inputs from the environment, other team members, the patient, and a multitude of other factors. This skill requires the abilities to obtain and comprehend information, as well as anticipate future events.[22]

### Decision Making

Good decision making is contingent on appropriate situational awareness. Once a situation is correctly understood, a judgment or decision often needs to be enacted. Decision making relies on a complex combination of cognitive strategies. Examples include the seemingly disparate strategies of rational analytical processes and intuitive pattern-recognition strategies. Rational analytical processes describes the ability to understand data (patient characteristics, medical literature, and so forth) to make a calculated decision based on data and facts. This type of thinking is linear, logical, and mathematical. Intuitive pattern recognition relies on experience, and pattern recognition guides decisions that make sense or "feel" right. Options must be considered, either implicitly or explicitly, and a decision must then be chosen, implemented, and reviewed for correctness.[22]

### Communication and Teamwork

Clear communication is essential to surgical safety, and breakdowns in communication lead to patient harm.[13–18] Communication can be verbal or nonverbal. Some basic principles of communication, such as learning and recalling the names of teammates in the operating room, enhance team dynamics and improve patient outcomes.[28] High-performing teams communicate clearly, exchange information effectively, establish mutual understanding, and coordinate care. This shared mental model facilitates efficient and effective teamwork, which makes operations safer.[22,29,30]

### Leadership

A broad field of study in itself, leadership includes the ability to galvanize people and coordinate all necessary actions in the service of a common vision. Leadership has been defined in several different ways, but, as it applies to the practice of surgery, it may be best understood in 3 parts as described by Pendleton and Furnham[31]: strategy, interpersonal traits, and operational implementation. Effective leadership in surgical practice leads to better quality and safety, an improved work environment, and efficient use of resources.[32] Leadership includes the ability to define and maintain standards, handle pressure, and support others.[22]

## TEACHING AND EVALUATING NONTECHNICAL SKILLS

The importance of nontechnical skills is now widely recognized. However, existing literature supporting a standardized approach or best practice for teaching and evaluating these skills is incomplete. Nontechnical skills are generally introduced and taught in a simulated operating room environment. Ongoing training and evaluation can occur in either a virtual or live setting. Training in a simulated operating room environment can involve high-fidelity simulation, low-fidelity simulation, crew (or crisis) resource management (CRM), and didactic sessions.[33]

High-fidelity simulation is a team-based activity in a simulated operating room environment to train nontechnical skills, usually to multiple leaners simultaneously. Existing data support the content, construct, and face validity of this model.[34] In addition, distributed simulation for high-fidelity simulation has been proposed, which uses a standardized high-fidelity model that is developed centrally and is then able to be transported/distributed to multiple training sites. Distributed simulation may reduce the cost, improve the ability to refine the model and training techniques, and gather more robust standardized data on the efficacy of the particular educational intervention. Simulation provides a safe environment for training as well as the capability for timely assessment and feedback.

Low-fidelity simulation often uses a less realistic environment or a component part of a simulated scenario, and may also be adequate and acceptable for trainees to learn nontechnical skills. When effective, low-fidelity scenarios have the benefits of being portable, more-cost effective, and more easily reproducible compared with high-fidelity models.[34] Although content, construct, and face validity of low-fidelity models have been shown, high-quality, comprehensive data supporting low-fidelity simulation are currently lacking.[33] More work needs to be done to determine whether high-fidelity models, with added complexity and cost, have any additional benefit to low-fidelity models.

CRM was developed in the 1980s by the aviation industry in response to several airline crashes caused by human error (communication lapses, poor decision making, failures in leadership).[35–37] The CRM program focuses on cockpit leadership, interpersonal communication, situation awareness, self-awareness, assertiveness, flexibility, adaptability, and decision making. CRM training comprises initial indoctrination/awareness, recurrence practice and feedback, and continual reinforcement. Functionally, CRM training combines aspects of didactics and simulation in ideal and complicated scenarios.[38] Like airplanes, operating rooms represent high-tech, high-risk environments subject to the same potential nontechnical failures that can lead to catastrophic outcomes.[12] This strategy makes intuitive sense and has shown benefit in aviation, but only a small number of low-quality studies exist to show benefit in a surgical context.[34] In addition, CRM training is often expensive and resource intensive.

Lecture formats to teach nontechnical skills have shown little to no benefit when studied in combination with other training modalities. Existing evidence does not support the use of didactics for training and evaluation of nontechnical skills. It seems that practice, either in live or simulated scenarios, confers skill acquisition and improvement.[39,40]

### Specific Training and Evaluation Tools

Training and evaluation tools for surgical nontechnical skills with validity and reliability data include Non-Technical Skills for Surgeons (NOTSS), Oxford Non-Technical Skills (NOTECHS and NOTECHS II), and Operative Observational Teamwork Assessment for Surgery (OTAS).[41]

NOTSS is a training course and behavior rating system developed to improve nontechnical surgical skills and provide reliable feedback regarding the skillset (the conceptual framework for NOTSS was constructed using a rigorous methodologic design and was described earlier). NOTSS can be used either in a simulated or live operating room environment. The NOTSS curriculum combines simulation and didactics using case-based scenarios. It has the most robust validity and reliability data of any existing curriculum, and has been tested using the OR Black Box system.[42–44] In addition, NOTSS also uses a rating scale including components corresponding with Accreditation Council for Graduate Medical Education (ACGME) core competencies. This model has been described as the gold-standard for individual assessment of nontechnical skills.[41] NOTSS has been adapted to the economic and cultural characteristics of several countries, including Rwanda, Denmark, the United States, and Japan.[5,26,45–47] Importantly, the evaluation tool is an individual performance assessment applied within a team context, which is unique among team-based evaluation tools.

In the Oxford NOTECHS[48–50] and the refined Oxford NOTECHS II[51] curricula, a trainer/observer evaluates the nontechnical skills of an entire surgical team in a live surgical situation. This process calculates a standardized numerical value that can be measured at various time intervals or after a significant intervention to assess improvement of nontechnical skills. This tool has good interrater reliability as well as construct and face validity, which have been demonstrated in multiple studies.[47–52] The NOTECHS II score more specifically measures nontechnical skills by removing confounders from technical performance.[51,52]

OTAS is a quantified scoring system that uses a Likert scale and generic checklist to assess communication, cooperation, coordination, shared leadership, team monitoring, and leadership in a live operating room. The evaluation is team based and can be useful when team members remain static over time.[42,53] OTAS uses a 7-point rating scale, compared with a 4-point scale for NOTECHS, and, therefore, may provide a more refined assessment of performance. Both the OTAS and NOTECHS tools assess team performance and operate under an assumption that teamwork is directly equivalent to a sum of component parts, the validity of which has not been tested.[54]

Other training and evaluation tools have been designed over the last 15 years, although there are currently few data regarding validation or reliability to support their use. The Mobile Mock Operating Room is a high-fidelity model using a simulated patient and operating room environment.[55] Participants reported the environment to be realistic and the model useful for building team dynamics. The Surgical Teamwork Tool measures surgical teamwork.[56] The 360° evaluation tool is a collaborative evaluation tool used by Harvard affiliated hospitals. This tool improved nontechnical skills in daily practice for 63% of participants. However, data on ability to generalize and validity are lacking.[57] The Metric for Evaluating Task Execution in the Operating Room was developed to measure intraoperative task completion for tasks relevant to successful surgical outcomes, and can identify gaps in nontechnical ability, but is not specifically designed to measure this domain.[58]

*Intraoperative Coaching*

Surgeons readily apply the idiom that practice makes perfect to technical skills in the OR, but they have not fully incorporated this notion into the practice of nontechnical skills. Deliberate practice and maintenance are important for consistent high performance of nontechnical skills. Surgical coaching has a demonstrated benefit in the improvement of technical skills.[59,60] Deliberate coaching of nontechnical skills is less commonly used but is equally effective in improvement of these skills over time. Min and colleagues[61] showed a medium effect size improvement in subjects who underwent coaching using the NOTSS framework, whereas controls in this study who did not receive coaching showed no improvement over time. Nontechnical skills may peak during fellowship training and fade with increasing time in practice.[62] This tendency may reflect lapses in team communication and sharing of information regarding decision making. Career-long coaching and professional development and assessment of nontechnical skills is necessary to improve patient outcomes.

## THE RISKS OF OVEREMPHASIZING NONTECHNICAL SKILLS

Despite the emphasis on nontechnical skills in this article, surgeons and hospital administrators must continue to teach and appreciate the technical aspects of surgery that are also crucial to good surgical outcomes. Overfocusing on nontechnical skills can ultimately detract from safe surgery because increased cognitive load can lead to poorer performance.[63] A study by Sexton and colleagues[64] evaluating nontechnical skills showed that improvement in simulation and communication enhances a team's anticipation (leading to decreased surgical times). However, this anticipation can lead to cognitive overload of surgical assistants, which may decrease situation awareness and compromise outcomes. In an editorial discussion of the Sexton and colleagues[64] study, Walle and Greenberg[65] suggest that maintaining an awareness of the limits of cognitive load, and minimizing inputs during key portions of an operation, may help avoid lapses in situation awareness and improve patient outcomes. Nontechnical skills are critical to quality care but must be understood as 1 component of surgical excellence that must be integrated with factors including knowledge base and technical proficiency to ensure excellent surgical outcomes and patient safety.

## FUTURE DIRECTIONS

The relationship between nontechnical surgical skills and patient outcomes is clear. Reliable, reproducible evaluative processes, including NOTSS, OTAS, and NOTECH II, are increasingly being used around the world. Although these models have been adapted to culture and socioeconomic differences in various countries, they are not yet widely enculturated into surgical training programs, maintenance of proficiency certifications, or institutional credentialing requirements. Surgical training programs should adopt curricula highlighting the importance of nontechnical surgical skills and teaching the fundamental tenets of leadership, situation awareness, teamwork, communication, and decision making. Whether using high-fidelity simulation or live operating environments, surgeons at all professional levels should be evaluated and held accountable for nontechnical excellence. Evidence of proficiency should be incorporated into institutional credentialing requirements.

## SUMMARY

Although sound, dexterous surgical technique is important, patient outcomes are inextricably linked to the nontechnical skills shown by the operating surgeon and the operative team. These cognitive, social, and behavioral skills, including leadership, communication, teamwork, situation awareness, and decision making, are critical components of the operating room environment; deficiencies in any of these areas can lead to significant complication or death. These skills can be learned. Several curricula have been developed for teaching and evaluating nontechnical skills. Given variation in social and behavioral norms in many countries, training tools may vary, but mastery of the skill set should be expected in all training programs and medical institutions in order to protect patients around the world. Validated assessment tools can be used to provide feedback in both simulated and real-life environments.

## DISCLOSURE

The authors have nothing to disclose.

## REFERENCES

1. Agha RA, Fowler AJ, Sevdalis N. The role of non-technical skills in surgery. Ann Med Surg (Lond) 2015;4(4):422–7.
2. Youngson GG. Teaching and assessing non-technical skills. Surgeon 2011; 9(Suppl1):S35–7.
3. Gawande AA, Zinner MJ, Studdert DM, et al. Analysis of errors reported by surgeons at three teaching hospitals. Surgery 2003;133(6):614–21.
4. Mazzocco K, Petitti DB, Fong KT, et al. Surgical team behaviors and patient outcomes. Am J Surg 2009;197(5):678–85.
5. Spanager L, Lyk-Jensen HT, Dieckmann P, et al. Customization of a tool to assess Danish surgeons' non-technical skills in the operating room. Dan Med J 2012; 59(11):A4526.
6. Weiser TG, Haynes AB, Molina G, et al. Estimate of the global volume of surgery in 2012: an assessment supporting improved health outcomes. Lancet 2015; 385(Suppl2):S11.
7. Densen P. Challenges and opportunities facing medical education. Trans Am Clin Climatol Assoc 2011;122:48–58.
8. Gawande A. Two hundred years of surgery. N Engl J Med 2012;367(6):582.
9. Kohn LT, Corrigan JM, Donaldson MS. Institute of Medicine (US) Committee on Quality Health Care in America. In: Kohn LT, Corrigan JM, Donaldson MS, editors. To err is human: building a safer health system. National Academies Press (US); 2000.
10. Donaldson L. An organisation with a memory. Clin Med (Lond) 2002;2(5):452–7.
11. Haynes AB, Weiser TG, Berry WR, et al. A surgical safety checklist to reduce morbidity and mortality in a global population. N Engl J Med 2009;360(5):491–9.
12. Klamen DL, Sanserino K, Skolnik P. Patient safety education: what was, what is, and what will be? Teach Learn Med 2013;25(sup1):S44–9.
13. Griffen FD, Stephens LS, Alexander JB, et al. The American College of Surgeons' closed claims study: new insights for improving care. J Am Coll Surg 2007; 204(4):561–9.
14. Greenberg CC, Regenbogen SE, Studdert DM, et al. Patterns of communication breakdowns resulting in injury to surgical patients. J Am Coll Surg 2007;204(4): 533–40.
15. Rogers SO Jr, Gawande AA, Kwaan M, et al. Analysis of surgical errors in closed malpractice claims at 4 liability insurers. Surgery 2006;140(1):25–33.

16. Lingard L, Espin S, Whyte S, et al. Communication failures in the operating room: an observational classification of recurrent types and effects. Qual Saf Health Care 2004;13(5):330–4.

17. Uramatsu M, Fujisawa Y, Mizuno S, et al. Do failures in non-technical skills contribute to fatal medical accidents in Japan? A review of the 2010–2013 national accident reports. BMJ Open 2017;7(2):e013678.

18. Scottish Audit of Surgical Mortality. Annual Report (2010). Available at: http://www.sasm.org.uk/Publications/Main.html. Accessed December 24, 2020.

19. Weiser TG, Regenbogen SE, Thompson KD, et al. An estimation of the global volume of surgery: a modelling strategy based on available data. Lancet 2008; 372(9633):139–44.

20. Chow A, Mayer EK, Darzi AW, et al. Patient-reported outcome measures: the importance of patient satisfaction in surgery. Surgery 2009;146(3):435–43.

21. Yule S, Flin R, Paterson-Brown S, et al. Non-technical skills for surgeons in the operating room: a review of the literature. Surgery 2006;139(2):140–9.

22. Yule S, Flin R, Paterson-Brown S, et al. Development of a rating system for surgeons' non-technical skills. Med Educ 2006;40(11):1098–104.

23. Flin R, Yule S, Paterson-Brown S, et al. Teaching surgeons about non-technical skills. Surgeon 2007;5(2):86–9.

24. Yule S, Flin R, Maran N, et al. Surgeons' non-technical skills in the operating room: reliability testing of the NOTSS behavior rating system. World J Surg 2008;32(4):548–56.

25. Yule S, Paterson-Brown S. Surgeons' non-technical skills. Surg Clin North Am 2012;92(1):37–50.

26. Yule S, Gupta A, Blair PG, et al. Gathering validity evidence to adapt the non-technical skills for surgeons (NOTSS) assessment tool to the United States context. J Surg Educ 2021;78(3):955–66.

27. Flin RH, O'Connor P, Crichton M. Safety at the sharp end: a guide to non-technical skills. Farnham (England): Ashgate Publishing, Ltd.; 2008.

28. Burton ZA, Guerreiro F, Turner M, et al. Mad as a hatter? Evaluating doctors' recall of names in theatres and attitudes towards adopting #theatrecapchallenge. Br J Anaesth 2018;121(4):984–6.

29. Birnbach DJ, Rosen LF, Fitzpatrick M, et al. Introductions during time-outs: do surgical team members know one another's names? Jt Comm J Qual Patient Saf 2017;43(6):284–8.

30. Mathieu JE, Heffner TS, Goodwin GF, et al. The influence of shared mental models on team process and performance. J Appl Psychol 2000;85(2):273–83.

31. Pendleton D, Furnham AF. Leadership: all you need to know. 2nd Edition. London (England): Springer; 2016.

32. Suliman A, Klaber RE, Warren OJ. Exploiting opportunities for leadership development of surgeons within the operating theatre. Int J Surg 2013;11(1):6–11.

33. Ounounou E, Aydin A, Brunckhorst O, et al. Nontechnical skills in surgery: a systematic review of current training modalities. J Surg Educ 2019;76(1):14–24.

34. Brewin J, Tang J, Dasgupta P, et al. Full immersion simulation: validation of a distributed simulation environment for technical and non-technical skills training in Urology. BJU Int 2015;116(1):156–62.

35. Diehl AE. Air safety investigators: using science to save lives—one crash at a time. Bloomington (IN): Xlibris Corporation; 2013.

36. Mckinney EH Jr, Barker JR, Davis KJ, et al. How swift starting action teams get off the ground: What United flight 232 and airline flight crews can tell us about team communication. Manag Commun Q 2005;19(2):198–237.

37. Helmreich RL, Merritt AC, Wilhelm JA. The evolution of crew resource management training in commercial aviation. Int J Aviat Psychol 1999;9(1):19–32.
38. AC 120-51E. Crew resource management training document information. Washington, DC: US Department of Transportation, FAA, Advisory Circular; 2004.
39. Dedy NJ, Bonrath EM, Ahmed N, et al. Structured training to improve nontechnical performance of junior surgical residents in the operating room. Ann Surg 2016;263(1):43–9.
40. Pena G, Altree M, Field J, et al. Nontechnical skills training for the operating room: a prospective study using and didactic workshop. Surgery 2015;158(1):300–9.
41. Wood TC, Raison N, Haldar S, et al. Training tools for nontechnical skills for surgeons—a systematic review. J Surg Educ 2017;74(4):548–78.
42. Whittaker G, Abboudi H, Khan MS, et al. Teamwork assessment tools in modern surgical practice: a systematic review. Surg Res Pract 2015;2015:494827.
43. Yule S, Gupta A, Gazarian D, et al. Construct and criterion validity testing of the Non-Technical Skills for Surgeons (NOTSS) behaviour assessment tool using videos of simulated operations. Br J Surg 2018;105(6):719–27.
44. Jung JJ, Yule S, Boet S, et al. Nontechnical skill assessment of the collective surgical team using the non-technical skills for surgeons (NOTSS) System. Ann Surg 2020;272(6):1158–63.
45. Lin Y, Scott JW, Mutabazi Z, et al. Strong support for a context-specific curriculum on non-technical skills for surgeons (NOTSS). East Cent Afr J Surg 2016; 21(3):3–5.
46. Scott JW, Lin Y, Ntakiyiruta G, et al. Identification of the critical nontechnical skills for surgeons needed for high performance in a variable-resource context (NOTSS-VRC). Ann Surg 2019;270(6):1070–8.
47. Tsuburaya A, Soma T, Yoshikawa T, et al. Introduction of the non-technical skills for surgeons (NOTSS) system in a Japanese Cancer Center. Surg Today 2016; 46(12):1451–5.
48. Mishra A, Catchpole K, Dale T, et al. The influence of non-technical performance on technical outcome in laparoscopic cholecystectomy. Surg Endosc 2008;22(1): 68–73.
49. Mishra A, Catchpole K, McCulloch P. The Oxford NOTECHS System: reliability and validity of a tool for measuring teamwork behaviour in the operating theatre. Qual Saf Health Care 2009;18(2):104–8.
50. McCulloch P, Mishra A, Handa A, et al. The effects of aviation-style non-technical skills training on technical performance and outcome in the operating theatre. Qual Saf Health Care 2009;18(2):109–15.
51. Robertson ER, Hadi M, Morgan LJ, et al. Oxford NOTECHS II: a modified theatre team non-technical skills scoring system. PLoS One 2014;9(3):e90320.
52. Robertson E, Morgan L, New S, et al. Quality improvement in surgery combining lean improvement methods with teamwork training: a controlled before-after study. PLoS One 2015;10(9):e0138490.
53. Hull L, Arora S, Aggarwal R, et al. The impact of nontechnical skills on technical performance in surgery: a systematic review. J Am Coll Surg 2012;214(2): 214–30.
54. Etherington N, Larrigan S, Liu H, et al. Measuring the teamwork performance of operating room teams: a systematic review of assessment tools and their measurement properties. J Interprof Care 2021;35(1):37–45.
55. Paige JT, Kozmenko V, Yang T, et al. High-fidelity, simulation-based, interdisciplinary operating room team training at the point of care. Surgery 2009;145(2): 138–46.

56. Huang LC, Conley D, Lipsitz S, et al. The surgical safety checklist and teamwork coaching tools: a study of inter-rater reliability. BMJ Qual Saf 2014;23(8):639–50.

57. Nurudeen SM, Kwakye G, Berry WR, et al. Can 360-degree reviews help surgeons? Evaluation of multisource feedback for surgeons in a multi-institutional quality improvement project. J Am Coll Surg 2015;221(4):837–44.

58. Russ S, Arora S, Wharton R, et al. Measuring safety and efficiency in the operating room: development and validation of a metric for evaluating task execution in the operating room. J Am Coll Surg 2013;216(3):472–81.

59. Gawande A. Top athletes and singers have coaches. Should you. New York: The New Yorker; 2011. p. 44–53.

60. Jule S, Parker SH, Wilkinson J, et al. Coaching Non-technical skills improves surgical residents' performance in a simulated operating room. J Surg Educ 2015; 72(6):1124–30.

61. Min H, Morales DR, Orgill D, et al. Systematic review of coaching to enhance surgeons' operative performance. Surgery 2015;158(5):1168–91.

62. Gostlow H, Marlow N, Thomas MJ, et al. Non-technical skills of surgical trainees and experienced surgeons. Br J Surg 2017;104(6):777–85.

63. Yurko YY, Scerbo MW, Prabhu AS, et al. Higher mental workload is associated with poorer laparoscopic performance as measured by the NASA-TLX tool. Simul Healthc 2010;5(5):267–71.

64. Sexton K, Johnson A, Gotsch A, et al. Anticipation, teamwork and cognitive load: chasing efficiency during robot-assisted surgery. BMJ Qual Saf 2018;27(2): 148–54.

65. Walle KV, Greenberg C. Intraoperative non-technical skills: a critical target for improving surgical outcomes. BMJ Qual Saf 2018;27(2):99–101.

# Intraoperative Teaching and Evaluation in General Surgery

Richard A. Sidwell, MD*

## KEYWORDS

- Operative teaching • Debriefing • Resident evaluation

## KEY POINTS

- Operative training is moving from a historically apprentice-based model to one based on defined objectives and measures of competence.
- Briefing before the operative procedure allows the instructor and trainee to agree on the educational goals to be achieved.
- Surgical teachers can learn best practices for intraoperative instruction through faculty development programs and feedback from learners.
- The Zwisch model describes operative progressive operative competence and autonomy and can be used as a summative feedback tool.
- OPRS and O-SCORE are effective tools for formative feedback of operative performance.

## INTRODUCTION

Learning to be a technically proficient surgeon, one who is competent for independent and unsupervised practice, is a core feature in the development of a general surgery resident. The domain of learning technical skills is a distinguishing feature of the surgical specialties and one that requires different strategies for teaching and learning than are needed for the domains of medical knowledge and clinical care. Historically this was accomplished through an apprentice-based model, where the surgical resident would spend extended periods of time in the operating room under the tutelage of an experienced surgeon. Resident confidence and autonomy were further developed while working with little or no supervision. This relatively unstructured approach to learning operative skills has given way to a modern approach that includes the use of simulation and skills training outside of the operating room and a movement toward objective measures of competence in the operating room. Still, as Dr Atul Gawande explained at the

Former Program Director of General Surgery Residency, Iowa Methodist Medical Center, Des Moines, IA, USA; Adjunct Clinical Professor, Department of Surgery, University of Iowa Carver College of Medicine, Iowa City, IA, USA
* Corresponding author. Department of Surgical Education, 1415 Woodland Avenue, Suite 140, Des Moines, IA 50309, USA.
*E-mail address:* rsidwell@iowaclinic.com

Surg Clin N Am 101 (2021) 587–595
https://doi.org/10.1016/j.suc.2021.05.006
0039-6109/21/© 2021 Elsevier Inc. All rights reserved.
surgical.theclinics.com

start of the twenty-first century, "Residency still largely relies on the wonderful, time-honored, throat-constricting method of learning-by-doing on-the-job training, as it were. It has worked for decades."[1] Indeed, the operating room remains the predominant and most important location where surgical residents learn operative judgment and technical skill. Although there are many ways to address the issue, this chapter seeks to succinctly present best practices regarding the specific aspects of surgical instruction—teaching and evaluation—that occur in the operating room.

## A FRAMEWORK FOR TEACHING IN THE OPERATING ROOM

Surgeons who are skilled in the operating room are not necessarily excellent instructors of surgical trainees. The traditional teaching model of "learning by doing" relies on the trainee eventually learning through the process of discovery; this requires volume of exposure rather than intentional teaching by the instructor. To address this realization, Roberts and colleagues introduced a model of intraoperative instruction-based "guided discovery," where the instructor provides preparatory information, intraoperative guidance, and postoperative feedback[2,3]; this is the B-I-D (Briefing, Intraoperative Teaching, Debriefing) model. A brief explanation and example of these components is as follows:

### Briefing

Briefing occurs before entering the operating room, perhaps even while scrubbing in preparation for the procedure. It is an opportunity for the teaching surgeon and the trainee to agree on the educational goals to be achieved during the operation. In educational terms, this is completion of a "needs assessment" and use of this information to articulate specific learning objectives for the procedure.

> *Briefing example #1:*
> *Surgeon*: "This is the first time that you've performed a hernia repair with me. What is your experience with this operation?"
> *Resident*: "I've read about the operation and studied the anatomy, but this is the first one that I've participated in."
> *Surgeon*: "OK. Let's review the key steps of the operation right now. As we work I want you to concentrate on these components."
> *Briefing example #2:*
> *Surgeon*: "Last week when you and I did a laparoscopic colectomy I noticed that you struggled with mobilization of the right colon."
> *Resident*: "Yes. I need to do a better job of using my left hand to create proper tension."
> *Surgeon*: "When we get to that portion of the operation, I'll demonstrate how I do it and then I'll specifically coach you with that maneuver."
> *Briefing example #3:*
> *Resident*: "I know that I can do this operation with you assisting and guiding me, but I don't know if I can direct someone else to be my assistant."
> *Surgeon*: "For this procedure, let's have the scrub tech assist you and I will observe and provide suggestions on how to better use your assistant."

This briefing establishes a common understanding between the instructor and learner regarding the educational expectations of the operation. It changes the experience from one of random discovery (teaching/learning based on whatever happens to occur in the procedure) to "guided discovery" (intentional teaching/learning of specific items based on the needs of the learner).

## Intraoperative Teaching

Intentional intraoperative instruction begins with the common understanding of the educational goals that were set out in the preoperative briefing. Although there are leaning opportunities throughout the operation, focus and emphasis is placed on these learning objectives. Timberlake and colleagues conducted a systematic review of the science regarding intraoperative teaching.[4] In this review, several studies were identified that provided a list of best instructional practices and themes. For example, Cox and Swanson[5] reported these qualities were associated with superior teaching in terms of resident evaluation:

- Demonstrating awareness and sensitivity to resident learning needs
- Providing direct and ongoing feedback regarding resident progress
- Demonstrating surgical technical expertise and up-to-date knowledge
- Allowing and encouraging resident participation in procedures
- Maintaining a supportive learning environment

This list of positive attributes of surgical teachers was expanded on in a report by Skoczylas and colleagues,[6] where 7 commonalities were identified:

- Emphasis on anatomic landmarks
- Supportive use of perceptual motor teaching (instructing learners to consider not only what they see but also what they feel)
- Encouragement of repetition
- Promotion of early independence
- Demonstration of confident competence (teaching surgeon is perceived as an expert who is competent to perform, teach, and handle complications)
- Calm demeanor in the operating room
- Willingness to accept responsibility for mistakes and its consequences

Putting this together, it would seem that the ideal surgical instructor is one who is confident and technically proficient, understands and encourages the learning needs of the trainee, teaches safe technique based on understanding of anatomy while providing useful feedback, maintains a supportive learning environment, and encourages development of the trainee's autonomy.

*Intraoperative teaching example #1:*
    *Surgeon*: "So, now that we have opened the fibers of the external oblique, what is the next step of this hernia repair?"
    *Resident*: "The spermatic cord needs to be mobilized."
    *Surgeon*: "Correct. Now I will show you how I do this and why I do it before dissecting the hernia sac free from the cord structures."
*Intraoperative teaching example #2:*
    *Surgeon*: "You have been efficient to this point. Now let me use the instruments briefly to show you how I use my left hand to create exposure and tension. See, I grasp on the tenia and pull toward the left side. Now you do it."
    *Resident*: Performs the maneuver correctly (with additional coaching as needed).
*Intraoperative teaching example #3:*
    *Surgeon*: Has been calmly sitting away from the operative field while the resident has been working to achieve a critical view of safety during a laparoscopic cholecystectomy, but the case is no longer progressing. "Don't assume that your assistant knows what you are trying to see and do." After briefly taking the instrument to show how the assistant can help expose, "Now, you show your assistant how to help you."

*Resident*: Practices teaching the assistant some helpful maneuvers to facilitate the operation.

Fortunately, surgical teachers can improve their intraoperative teaching skill through faculty development exercises and feedback from their learners. Gardner and colleagues developed and reported on the effectiveness of an intraoperative teaching course for surgeons.[7] This 4-hour activity taught the framework of the Briefing, Intraoperative Teaching, Debriefing model, concluding with a teaching exercise in a virtual operating room setting. When participating faculty surgeons were evaluated 2 months after the education exercise, teaching behavior was noted to be improved, *especially among those who started in the lowest quartile*. Not surprisingly, the experienced and skilled instructors did not have the same improvement; this shows that faculty development programs can be effective in improving the overall teaching quality to which the trainees are exposed.

### Debriefing

Immediately following the operation, the teaching surgeon and the trainee should debrief about the procedure and the specific learning objectives. As described by Roberts, "The debriefing consists of 4 elements: reflection, rules, reinforcement, and correction."[2]

*Reflection*: the teaching surgeon asks the trainee for a self-assessment of what was learned in relation to the identified learning objective. It is important for the instructor to understand the insight that the learner has into their performance.
*Rules*: the trainee should articulate the specific learning points that have been acquired during the operation.
*Reinforcement*: the teaching surgeon reiterates and reinforces the things that were done correctly, especially as related to the learning objectives.
*Correction*: correcting any mistakes that were made is necessary in order to prevent these mistakes from recurring; this should include not only *what* was wrong but also *why* it was wrong and *how* to do it correctly the next time.

The process of the debrief does not need to take long, no more than several minutes; this can be done while still in the operating room (while closing, for example) or immediately after leaving the room. It should be conducted promptly while the learning objectives and intraoperative instruction are fresh in the minds of the instructor and the learner.

*Debriefing example (for scenario #3)*:
*Surgeon*: "What did you learn about making use of your assistant?"
*Resident*: "It was hard at first because I assumed that they would know how to help me. It did get easier as I practiced. I learned that I need to show the assistant what I'm trying to see and clearly explain how to help me a little better."
*Surgeon*: "Yes, it is harder when you are working with someone who isn't familiar with you or with the operation. You need to teach them the specific things you want. Be careful – I could see you had some frustration. Keep that under control or it will undo the collegial environment that you are creating."

Although feedback and debriefing are essential components of intraoperative instruction, surgical instructors do not always do it very well. Ahmed and colleagues conducted a 2-part study to evaluate surgical debriefings.[8] First teachers and learners were queried regarding features of effective debriefing. Then, surgical cases were observed to determine how closely the actual debriefing reflected the identified optimal practices. **Table 1** presents a comparison of the optimal and observed practices. Trainees and trainers indicated that optimal debriefing would occur both during and after the operative procedure; this allows immediate correction of errors and reinforcement of correct actions. Most of the participants also agreed that debriefing should be structured around the stated learning objectives and should include areas that went well and those that did not.

The observed practices fell short of the optimal behavior. The debriefing and feedback was done verbally in an unstructured fashion during the procedure without being related to defined learning objectives. Positive feedback was seen, but it was nonspecific in nature ("There you go, well done"). Most of the observed feedback was correctional in nature but was without identification of specific strategies for improvement. Finally, the debriefing was observed to be related only to technical factors, not nontechnical issues such as teamwork and communication. This study presents a clear opportunity for faculty development in terms of effective debriefing.

## EVALUATION OF OPERATIVE PERFORMANCE

The process of evaluation of a trainee's operative performance has also undergone transformation in the twenty-first century. Previously, faculty evaluation of a resident's progress and capability was akin to Supreme Court Justice Potter Stewart's words in his concurring opinion in *Jacobellis vs. Ohio (1964)*, where he wrote "I shall not today attempt further to define the kind of material I understand to be embraced within that shorthand description; and perhaps I could never succeed in intelligibly doing so. But *I know it when I see it*…"[9] This approach may have been effective in decades past, but it neglects the modern concept of progressive autonomy based on documented competence. Every surgical residency program has developed and tried multiple methods of operative evaluation. Presented here are some best practice examples.

### The Zwisch Model

Named for its originator, Dr Joseph Zwischenberger, the Zwisch model is a simple method of assessing residents in the operating room.[10] It consists of 4 stages of progressive operative development and autonomy. These stages are shown in **Fig. 1**.

> *Show and tell*: the trainee is the first assistant and an active observer of the operation. The teaching surgeon performs the key portions while demonstrating techniques, anatomy, etc. In addition, the teaching surgeon verbalizes the important steps and concepts through the operation.

**Table 1**
**Comparison of optimal and observed debriefing practice**

|  | Optimal Debriefing Practice | Observed Debriefing Practice |
|---|---|---|
| Approach and timing of debriefing | Structured debriefing done during and immediately after the operative procedure | Unstructured debriefing done only during the operative procedure, focusing on corrective action |
| Content of debriefing | Focus on positive and negative aspects of performance, including technical and nontechnical skills, with specific strategies to improve performance | Nonspecific positive feedback, with most feedback being negative and focused on technical skills, without a plan for improvement |

*Adapted from* Ahmed, and colleagues[8]

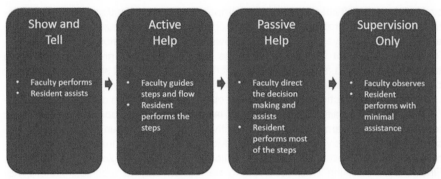

**Fig. 1.** Zwisch scale of progressive operative competence and autonomy. (*Adapted from* DaRosa, et al.[10]).

*Active (a.k.a. "smart") help*: the trainee and teaching surgeon alternate between the operating and first assistant roles in the operation. The teaching surgeon, when assisting, actively leads the trainee through exposure and coaching.

*Passive (a.k.a. "dumb") help*: the trainee now progresses through the operation with increasing efficiency. The teaching surgeon provides assistance while following the lead of the trainee. Coaching is primarily limited to help with decision-making.

*Supervision only (a.k.a. "no help")*: the trainee performs the operation without assistance from the teaching surgeon, using operating room staff or junior trainees as assistants. The teaching surgeon monitors the progress of the operation and continues to assure patient safety.

The Zwisch model is a simple and logical construct for development of operative skills and progressive autonomy. It is also easily translated into a "scale" that can be used to provide feedback regarding resident performance in the operating room.[11] George and colleagues used a novel "smart phone" application to request and record an evaluation of the trainee's performance immediately after every operation, ultimately collecting 1490 evaluations on 31 residents from 27 faculty surgeons. The scale was found to have construct validity in that the amount of faculty guidance decreased and the level of resident autonomy increased according to advancing postgraduate year (PGY) of the resident. The scale was also found to correlate with the operative performance of the trainee. Finally, interrater agreement was high, demonstrating reliability of this simple scale. Moreover, teaching faculty can easily learn to use the Zwisch scale in as little as a 1-hour faculty development session.[12]

One drawback of the Zwisch scale is that it is a global assessment of the trainee's operative performance and autonomy. It does not evaluate the specific individual components of intraoperative competency. Thus, its best use may be for summative rather than formative evaluation. To achieve the granularity necessary for formative evaluation, a different evaluative tool may be necessary.

### Operative Performance Ratings System and Ottawa Surgical Competency Operating Room Evaluation

The teaching faculty at Southern Illinois University developed the Operative Performance Ratings System (OPRS) in 2001.[13] Initially paper-based and then converted to an electronic format distributed by a residency management system, this system selected 2 operations that represented typical and common procedures for each PGY level (PGY-1 through PGY-5). A 10-item instrument that focused on procedure-specific skills and decisions was then created that was specific for each operation. The teaching surgeon would evaluate the trainee's performance on each item using a scale of 1 ("very poor") to 5 ("clearly superior"). **Fig. 2** shows an example OPRS used at the author's institution, which was adapted directly from that developed and published by Larsen and colleagues.[13] The OPRS was found to be an effective method of evaluating resident performance, and data collection was easier once switching from a paper to an electronic platform.

One drawback of the OPRS is that the rated items are specific to an individual procedure, meaning that a separate evaluation tool would need to be developed for all procedures for which evaluative feedback is desired. To address this, Gofton and colleagues developed the Ottawa Surgical Competency Operating Room Evaluation (O-SCORE).[14] O-SCORE is a succinct assessment tool that can be used for any operative procedure. As finalized, it consisted of 8 items rated on a 5-point scale (with anchoring language), 1 yes/no question, and 2 open-ended questions. Items rated included

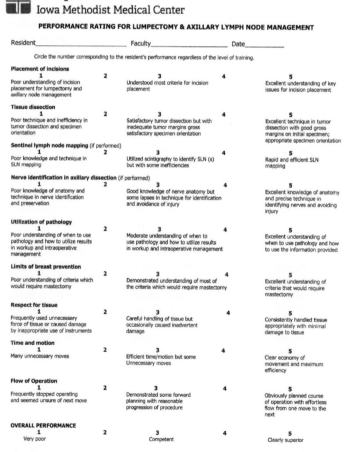

**Fig. 2.** Sample OPRS evaluation form used at the author's institution. (*Adapted from* Larson and colleagues[13]).

1. Preprocedure plan
2. Case preparation
3. Knowledge of specific procedural steps
4. Technical performance
5. Visuospatial skills
6. Postprocedure plan
7. Efficiency and flow
8. Communication

The teaching surgeon also completed these queries:

- Resident is able to safely perform *this* procedure *independently* (Yes/No)
- Give at least 1 *specific* aspect of the procedure done well (open-ended)
- Give at least 1 *specific* suggestion for improvement (open-ended)

The O-SCORE tool was found to be useful and practical for both teaching surgeons and trainees. Teaching surgeons found it easy to use. Residents found the assessments to clearly indicate where improvements were necessary in order to achieve competence.

The best practice for evaluating operative performance is still developing. The ideal method needs to be valid and reliable, easy-to-use by teachers and trainees, and able to provide information that can be used in both formative and summative manners. Achieving this specific, timely, and consistent feedback is a challenge for residency programs. Innovative, technology-based solutions are being explored[15,16] but have yet to achieve broad penetration.

## SUMMARY

For the surgical resident, the operating room remains the primary location for learning technical skills and the nontechnical requirements (decision-making, communication, team leadership) of a competent surgeon. The process of this education is in a state of evolution in the twenty-first century. In the past, competence was achieved in somewhat of a "brute force" manner. This relied on heavy operative exposure and unsupervised trainee experiences. The climate of surgical education has changed, so, too, is the manner in which intraoperative instruction occurs. It is now recognized that trainee learning is most efficient when "guided discovery," based on predefined educational needs and learning objectives and reinforced by brief postprocedural feedback, is used. As demonstrated in this chapter, this process is not an arduous one. Surgical instructors can easily learn and incorporate the B-I-D model of intraoperative instruction through faculty development exercises. Evaluation and feedback of operative performance is also undergoing changes. Again, there are effective models (Zwisch) and tools (OPRS, O-SCORE), although the optimal methods of using them are still being investigated. It is likely that use of technology will allow improved data collection that can be used for both formative and summative feedback, allowing advancement of surgical residents to be competency-based.

## DISCLOSURE

The author has nothing to disclose.

## REFERENCES

1. Gawande A. Creating the educated surgeon in the 21st Century. Am J Surg 2001; 181:551–6.

2. Roberts NK, Williams RG, Kim M, et al. The briefing, intraoperative teaching, de-briefing model for teaching in the operating room. J Am Coll Surgeons 2009; 208(2):299–303.
3. Wood JD, Poola P, Mellinger JD. Effective intraoperative teaching: from theory to practice, RISE (Resources in Surgical Education), American College of Surgeons Division of Education. 2020. Available at: https://www.facs.org/education/division-of-education/publications/rise/articles/intraoperative-teaching. Accessed January 15, 2021.
4. Timberlake MD, Mayo H, Scott L, et al. What do we know about intraoperative teaching? Ann Surg 2017;266(2):251–9.
5. Cox SS, Swanson M. Identification of teaching excellence in operating room and clinic settings. Am J Surg 2002;183:251–5.
6. Skoczylas LC, Littleton EB, Kanter SL, et al. Teaching techniques in the operating room: the importance of perceptual motor teaching. Acad Med 2012;87(3): 364–71.
7. Gardner AK, Timberlake MD, Dunkin BJ. Faculty development for the operating room: an examination of the effectiveness of an intraoperative teaching course for surgeons. Ann Surg 2019;269(1):184–90.
8. Ahmed M, Sevdalis N, Vincent C, et al. Actual vs perceived performance debrief-ing in surgery: practice far from perfect. Am J Surg 2013;205(4):434–40.
9. Brennan WJ & Supreme Court Of The United States. US Reports: Jacobellis v. Ohio, 378 U.S. 184. [Periodical] Retrieved from the Library of Congress, 1963. Available at: https://www.loc.gov/item/usrep378184/
10. DaRosa DA, Zaischenberger JB, Meyerson SL, et al. A theory-based model for teaching and assessing residents in the operating room. J Surg Educ 2013; 70(1):24–30.
11. George BC, Teitelbaum EN, Meyerson SL, et al. Reliability, validity, and feasibility of the zwisch scale for the assessment of intraoperative performance. J Surg Educ 2014;71(6):e90–6.
12. George BC, Teitelbaum EN, DaRosa DA, et al. Duration of faculty training needed to ensure reliable OR performance ratings. J Surg Educ 2013;70(6):703–8.
13. Larson JL, Williams RG, Ketchum J, et al. Feasibility, reliability and validity of an operative performance ratings system for evaluating surgery residents. Surgery 2005;183(4):640–9.
14. Gofton WT, Dudek NL, Wood TJ, et al. The Ottawa Surgical Competency Oper-ating Room Evaluation (O-SCORE): a tool to assess surgical competence. Acad Med 2012;87(10):1401–7.
15. Bohnen JD, George BC, Williams RG, et al, Procedural Learning and Safety Collaborative (PLSC). The feasibility of real-time intraoperative performance assessment with SIMPL (System for Improving and Measuring Procedural Learning): early experience from a multi-institutional trial. J Surg Educ 2016; 73(6):e118–30.
16. Karim AS, Sternback JM, Bender EM, et al. Quality of operative performance feedback given to thoracic surgery residents using an app-based system. J Surg Educ 2017;74(6):e81–7.

# General Surgery Resident Autonomy: Truth and Myth

Jason W. Kempenich, MD*, Daniel L. Dent, MD

## KEYWORDS

- Resident autonomy • General surgery • Confidence • Patient ownership

## KEY POINTS

- There is great concern that resident autonomy is not provided in sufficient quantity to fulfill the education needs for adequate general surgery training.
- Resident autonomy is likely most important for optimal learning, development of surgeon confidence, and appropriate ownership of patient outcomes.
- Barriers to autonomy include concerns of the general public and patients, regulatory constraints, and educational factors.

## INTRODUCTION

Within general surgery education circles, the state of autonomy for residents in surgery training programs has been of growing concern.[1–3] Although there is no direct objective evidence supporting that there is less autonomy in modern surgical training, multiple surrogates have been cited as reasons for concern. First, the American College of Surgeons created the Transition to Practice Fellowship in 2013 (renamed the Mastery of Surgery Fellowship) with one of the primary purposes being to "help fill the perceived gaps in training today," with the first goal being to "obtain enhanced autonomous experience in broad-based general surgery."[4] Second, greater than 80% of general surgery residents pursue fellowship after general surgery training,[5] which has led many to question whether the reason so many general surgery residency graduates pursue fellowship is that they lack the confidence to practice independently.[6,7] Third, multiple published articles link the perception of degraded resident confidence and patient ownership as symptoms of decreased autonomy.[2,6,8–10] Many reasons have been given for lost autonomy, including the 80-hour work week,[5] financial constraints,[11,12] concerns over quality of patient care,[13] patient expectations,[10,14] new and innovative technologies,[5] legal limitations,[15] and public opinion.[16,17]

UT Health San Antonio, Department of Surgery, 7703 Floyd Curl Drive, San Antonio, TX 78229-3900, USA
* Corresponding author.
E-mail address: kempenich@uthscsa.edu

Surg Clin N Am 101 (2021) 597–609
https://doi.org/10.1016/j.suc.2021.05.007
0039-6109/21/© 2021 Elsevier Inc. All rights reserved.

## THE CURRENT STATE OF AUTONOMY

The Libby Zion case occurred in 1984 and has been cited as a major event that has led to regulatory changes in postgraduate medical education. In short, a young woman died in the hospital 6 hours after being admitted by a junior resident and the patient had not been seen by a faculty physician. After investigation, multiple recommendations were made by a New York Grand Jury and subsequently the Bell Commission that have materialized into our modern Accreditation Council for Graduate Medical Education (ACGME) work hours restrictions and supervision requirements.[16] Griner and colleagues[8] conducted a survey of attending faculty comparing impressions of residents trained under work hour restrictions compared with residents trained before the 80-hour work week. Eighty percent of attending faculty thought that those residents who were trained under the 80-hour work week were less ready to operate independently and 66% trusted the residents less to care for patients. Teman and colleagues[10] also reported that teaching faculty thought that, compared with their own training, current residents had less operating room autonomy, residents were not as prepared to operate independently, and there was more need for fellowship training. This perspective seemed to further be cemented with the publication of the often-quoted survey of fellowship directors by Mattar and colleagues[3] in which they report that 70% of fellowship directors would trust a fellow to perform a laparoscopic cholecystectomy and only 34% would trust a fellow to perform 30 minutes of a major operation without supervision.

Napolitano and colleagues[2] published a survey comparing impressions from those surgeons more than 45 years old and those less than 45 years old. Almost all junior surgeons (93.6%) thought they were adequately trained to transition to the role of attending surgeon. In contrast, only 53% of surgeons more than 45 years old thought that junior surgeons were adequately prepared to take on the role of attending surgeon. Junior surgeons estimated that on average they called on senior surgeons for assistance approximately 10% of the time. However, 50% of senior surgeons reported that they assisted junior surgeons with 10% to 40% of procedures. Interestingly, when junior surgeons were asked why they pursued fellowship training, none reported, "Because I didn't think I was ready to practice."

Of note, psychologists have studied the concept of generational bias, the belief that one's own generation is superior to others. They have found that bias does exist and that stereotypes that spur bias are rarely accurate.[18] All the studies cited earlier are potentially subject to such bias.

This disparity in perception of training also carries over when comparing perspectives of appropriate levels of autonomy between faculty and residents. Both general surgery faculty and residents believe that chief residents need a significant amount of autonomy, but, in comparison, residents consistently rate the level of autonomy higher than faculty ($P = .003$).[17] In a survey of anesthesiology attendings and residents evaluating entrustable professional activities (EPAs), residents report performing EPAs at higher levels than faculty expect.[19] This effect is most pronounced in the earlier years of training. This discrepancy disappears with chief-level residents and there is agreement between faculty and residents. The investigators suggested that overconfidence may be necessary to optimize learning; that is, if trainees do not think they can accomplish a task, they may be less likely to try. Regardless, in a survey administered to all general surgery residents along with the 2008 American Board of Surgery In-Service Training Examination, 26% of those surveyed worried they would not be confident to operate independently on graduation.[6] Those who worried about operating independently were more likely to think that fellowship was required after general surgery residency ($P<.001$).

Lewis and Klingensmith[5] appropriately point out in their article detailing issues in general surgery training that the principal change in general surgery training over the last few decades is the conversion of many operations to laparoscopic techniques from open procedures. This change only continues to increase with the advent and increasing adoption of laparoscopic procedures using robotic platforms. They go on to define how advances in endoscopic treatment of biliary stone disease, endovascular treatment of vascular disease, as well as improved computed tomography resolution and diagnostic capability in patients with trauma have all been technological advancements that have changed the general surgery resident training experience as well as the practice of general surgery. Others have suggested that the need for further fellowship training is the natural effect of continued technological innovation and complexity and that solid general surgery training in combination with specialized skill acquisition through fellowship should be embraced.[20,21]

At present, The best measures of autonomy come from survey data citing surrogates for autonomy and best recollection. In 1 survey, faculty and residents were in agreement across 3 institutions: 62% and 53%, respectively, thought the current resident autonomy level was appropriate.[17] Those who thought there was too little or far too little autonomy were 38% and 47%, respectively. No one surveyed thought that residents had too much autonomy (**Fig. 1**). This study included programs from the southern United States and the Midwest. Efforts are underway through a recent survey administered along with the ABSITE to further characterize chief resident operative independence across surgical training in the United States.

## WHY IS AUTONOMY IMPORTANT?

The Halstead method for surgery resident education has been successfully training surgeons for more than 100 years.[5,22] The Halstead method as well as the ACGME program requirements for Graduate Medical Education in General Surgery iterate a path for increasing supervised independence of residents over time commensurate with their competence levels.[23] Self-determination theory states that human beings naturally develop toward autonomous behavior, and, when they act autonomously, they learn better and achieve superior performance.[24] General surgery training has been built on a foundation of progressive independence. In a survey of residents,

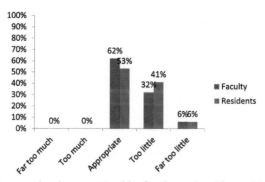

**Fig. 1.** Current autonomy level as perceived by faculty and residents. (*Adapted from* Kempenich JW, Willis RE, Rakosi R, Wiersch J, Schenarts PJ. How do perceptions of autonomy differ in general surgery training between faculty, senior residents, hospital administrators, and the general public? A multi-institutional study. Journal of Surgical Education. 2015;72(6):e193-e201; with permission).

faculty, and administrators, all 3 groups thought autonomy was important in surgical training (98%, 97%, 95%, respectively).[17]

### Struggle and Skill Acquisition

Supporting this idea that autonomy is important for surgical training, Willis and colleagues[25] recently published an article showing that when novices struggle first with a technical skill, they achieved superior performance. In medical students, 2 groups were assigned after seeing a demonstration of laparoscopic intracorporeal knot tying. The first were given instruction on the task, then pretested, practiced, and posttested. The second group pretested first, then were given instruction on the task, practiced, and posttested. **Fig. 2** shows that the group that struggled first with the task and were then given instruction achieved superior performance on the posttest. This theme of struggle as an important aspect to technical skill acquisition also emerged from a recent qualitative study examining factors that led to resident entrustment and autonomy through a semistructured interview of residents and faculty.[26]

Keeping in mind that safe struggle is desirable for better learning, Chen and colleagues[27] evaluated the perception of guidance provided to residents by faculty. To do this, they recorded procedures in which faculty had evaluated the residents as well as the level of guidance they provided to the resident. Expert raters then reviewed those videos and assigned their own rating of resident performance as well as level of guidance afforded to the resident by the teaching faculty. They found that most teaching faculty underestimate the level of guidance provided. In a follow-up study comparing resident and faculty perception of guidance in the operating room, faculty identified guidance 91.4% of the time compared with residents who only detected guidance 61.25% of the time.[28] Both of these articles point to the difficulty teaching faculty have in allowing safe struggle. Faculty may underestimate the help they give, and residents do not recognize at times when extra assistance is being rendered. This difficulty likely also clouds the ability of faculty and residents to assess trainee competence. In an effort to address these concerns, the American Board of Surgery has started the EPA pilot project in an effort to assess competency and performance.[29]

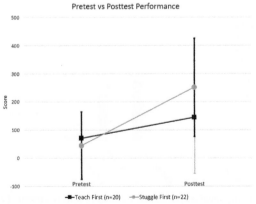

**Fig. 2.** The struggle-first group had a lower pretest score but achieved superior performance on the posttest. (*From* Willis RE, Erwin D, Adelaja F. Struggling Prior to a Teaching Even Results in Superior Short-Term Skills Acquisition in Novice Learners. Journal of Surgical Education. 2020;77(1):34–9; with permission).

## Confidence

Autonomy has been strongly linked by many to trainee confidence.[5,6,12,17,30,31] In 1 survey across multiple institutions, 94% of faculty and 92% of residents agreed or strongly agreed that more autonomy leads to increased self-confidence.[17] In a survey of surgeons evaluating characteristics required for managing and intervening during critical situations, confidence was listed #2 in the top 5 characteristics behind compe-tence and preceding composure, preparation, and experience.[32] Both surgery and medicine residents value the ability to make independent decisions to increase confi-dence.[31] Chalabian and Bremner[12] describe the importance of confidence to resident surgeons as equivalent to surgical self-efficacy, defined as the "...ability to organize and execute all of the necessary decision making and technical steps to complete a surgical procedure at a desired level of performance..." This definition of self-efficacy is closely aligned to the development of trust between faculty and resident. Olle ten Cate[33] states that trust is created when a competent trainee executes a task when appropriate to do so, and this is also a definition for performance. Putting it all together, competent performance leads to both trust and confidence.

The question then becomes, if trainees are confident, does that mean they are competent? Most surgeons have been acquainted with both trainees and/or col-leagues who potentially express more confidence than their competence seems to warrant. These anecdotal experiences are supported by multiple studies published in the literature. Sterkenburg and colleagues[19] showed that anesthesia junior residents were prone to overconfidence. Leopold and colleagues[34] similarly showed that, among practitioners attending a continuing medical education session on knee injec-tion, before instruction those who were most confident were the least competent ($P = .02$). After instruction, competence and confidence were more appropriately aligned ($P = .04$). Hassett and colleagues[35] showed that, when evaluating residents' history-taking skills and interpersonal skills using standardized patients for evaluation, confidence grows without similar improvement in performance. Other studies have shown that postgraduate year (PGY) 2 and PGY3 residents seem to experience a lull or even a decrease in confidence compared with their PGY1 year, with improve-ments as they progress to later years in training and early career as faculty.[6,19,31]

The explanation for the increase, decrease, and recovery of confidence through training and a surgeon's early career may be found in the psychology literature in the landmark article entitled, "Unskilled and Unaware of It: How Difficulties in Recog-nizing One's Own Incompetence Lead to Inflated Self-Assessments." Kruger and Dunning[36] performed 4 experiments in college students evaluating the interplay of confidence and competence using a humor proficiency test, a logical reasoning test, and a grammar test. There were 3 main conclusions. First, those who performed in the lowest quartile overestimated their performance, rating themselves as better than average. They scored in the 12th percentile on the humor test (similar results for the logic test), whereas they estimated that they performed in the 58th percentile ($P<.001$). Except for the top quartile, most participants overestimated their ability, but not to the same degree as the bottom quartile. The top quartile perceived their ability to be at the 72nd percentile but performed at the 89th ($P<.05$; **Fig. 3**). Second, when provided feedback on performance in the form of comparison of subjects' test to peers, self-assessment did not improve for the bottom quartile. Subjects in the bottom quartile thought they did even better than they originally thought after reviewing others' performance, suggesting that, in this group, feedback alone fails. By contrast, those in the top quartile estimated their ability more accurately with feedback. Third, with training, those in the bottom quartile recalibrated to a much more accurate

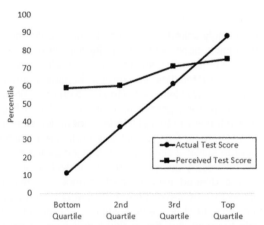

**Fig. 3.** Perceived ability to recognize humor compared with actual test performance. (*From* Kruger J, Dunning D. Unskilled and Unaware of It: How Difficulties in Recognizing One's Own Incompetence Lead to Inflated Self-Assessments. Journal Of Personality and Social Psychology. 1999;77(6):1121–34; with permission).

assessment of their performance. However, they still thought themselves to be performing better than their actual percentile. Those in the top quartile also recalibrated and seemed to understand their expertise better. This finding underscores the value of teaching to both novice and more experienced trainees.

In summary, the data regarding confidence reveal that, although autonomy is likely important for evaluation of performance and the development of confidence, measurement of confidence is a very poor surrogate to evaluate performance and autonomy, supported by both the medical education and the psychology literature. Operative autonomy is likely important to assess performance given the difficulties in allowing safe struggle presented earlier. However, the variability in confidence and factors that contribute indicate that measurement of confidence among trainees for the purpose of drawing conclusions about autonomy are inappropriate.

### Patient Ownership

Patient ownership is defined by Randel and colleagues[9] as the "clinicians' deep sense of responsibility for their patient's care and outcomes." Autonomy has often been cited as a key factor in the development of patient ownership in trainees.[9,10,17,30] Autonomy in resident training has been defined by Hinchey and colleagues[30] as "both patient ownership and the active direction of one's own learning." Similar to confidence, when autonomy decreased, 92% of faculty and 100% of residents thought that patient ownership decreased.[17] After implementation of the 80-hour work week, faculty have thought that patient ownership has markedly worsened.[8] In addition, surgery faculty endorse that they provide less autonomy when residents lack ownership.[10]

Randle and colleagues[9] explored the idea of patient ownership in surgical training across multiple institutions. Using a psychological ownership scale, residents who scored higher on the ownership scale reported greater satisfaction with the autonomy allowed by their residency programs ($P = .03$). Residents and faculty also agreed that increased operative autonomy also led to increased resident ownership. Despite this, only 53.7% of faculty granted more autonomy to increase resident sense of ownership. By contrast, 97.8% of faculty granted more autonomy to residents who show a strong sense of ownership. This finding is in line with faculty behavior as reported by Teman and colleagues[10] Both residents and faculty agreed that making the decision to operate created the greatest sense of patient ownership in residents. Development of patient ownership and the sense of responsibility required of surgeons cannot be overlooked. Autonomy seems to play a key role in developing this ethos.

### Struggle, Confidence, and Ownership

Surgical training in the United States has been built with autonomy as a cornerstone in the development of residents into independent practicing surgeons. Autonomy is necessary to allow optimal learning, assessment of trainee progress, as well as the development of confidence and patient ownership within the trainees.

## BARRIERS TO RESIDENT AUTONOMY

Multiple factors have been implicated when evaluating loss of resident autonomy. These factors can be understood in 3 main categories: concerns of the general public and patients, regulatory constraints, and educational factors.

### Concerns of the Public and Patients

Multiple studies have shown that, in general, patients and the general public are willing to have residents involved in their care (80%–95% acceptance).[14,17,37–41] Although this is encouraging, surgery has some unique challenges when gaining patient assent for resident involvement with surgical procedures. The general public and patients tend to be more comfortable with more experienced residents under supervision of the attending.[17,37,39,40,42] Dickinson and colleagues[39] reported that almost a third of respondents would not allow a resident to perform an operation on them without the attending in the room. This finding is similar to another study of the general public that revealed only 73% of respondents would consent for a routine procedure to be performed independently by a chief resident.[17] Another survey performed in an academic center solicited comfort levels of patients and their family members on the day of surgery with different portions of the operation.[42] They found that patients were comfortable with resident participation for all portions of surgery if the attending was present. Comfort level decreased if the attending was not present in the operating room for all steps, including prepping and positioning as well as closing the incision.

The general public also has concerns that resident involvement may lead to increased risk of complication.[39] Comparing perceptions of quality of care between residents, faculty, and administrators, they all agree that residents have a positive effect, whereas most of the general public believe there is no impact.[17] The literature regarding outcomes associated with resident involvement is largely mixed, with some studies showing an increased risk of complication[43–45] and others showing no effect,[46–48] and some showing increased risk of complication but lower risk of mortality.[49] On a positive note, in a survey of faculty surgeons, most surgeons thought they were able assuage patient concerns to allow trainee participation.[50]

### Regulatory Constraints

The 2 most significant regulatory events that are pointed to as potential root causes for the loss of resident autonomy are the 80-hour work week[5] and the revision to published rules for the payment of services of teaching physicians that stipulated the attending surgeon was required to be present for the key portions of a procedure in order to bill for services rendered by residents.[12]

The effect of the 80-hour work week as perceived by multiple surveys was discussed earlier when evaluating the current state of autonomy.[2,5,8] Early perception was that the limitations on duty hours decreased overall time to train and acquire experience before graduation and independent practice.[5] This perception was objectively noted by Kairys and colleagues[51] when significant reductions in first assistant (77%) and teaching assistant (66%) cases were seen in national resident case logs. This reduction of hours in the hospital and in the operating room was also perceived to negatively affect the culture of general surgery training.[8] The limitation for most of these data is that they are based on perception and recollection. Other confounding factors, such as changes to regulations on reimbursement as well as changing technology (eg, laparoscopic surgery), are temporally related to the advent of work hour restrictions. All these confounding factors limit the current ability to draw larger conclusions about the 80-hour work week and its effect on autonomy for general surgery residents.

Regulations on reimbursement have largely increased the demand for attending presence in the operating room. In Chalabian and Bremner's[12] report discussing the effect of government policy requiring attending surgeon presence for reimbursement of services from 1998, they cite that residents find attending presence in the operating room detrimental. Teman and colleagues,[10] in their survey of surgery faculty evaluating perceptions of barriers to resident operative autonomy, found that most faculty did not believe productivity targets had a significant impact on resident autonomy. Interestingly, those faculty who trained before work hour restrictions were more likely to believe such regulations detrimental to operative autonomy. They also found that faculty did not believe risk of litigation to be of significant impact. In another study, 70% of faculty agreed that regulations regarding reimbursement decreased autonomy and, again, this effect was more pronounced in those faculty with more than 10 years of teaching experience.[17]

Although some evidence points to faculty belief that such regulations are detrimental to resident autonomy, there are multiple studies reviewing the effect of supervision on patient care. When evaluated objectively, multiple studies find that more supervision of residents leads to improved patient care and educational outcomes.[52,53] When examining medical expertise, it is theorized that physician experts draw on mental models created by experiences with multiple prior patients.[54] This theory may explain the importance of attending oversight to patient care and educational outcomes. The hurdle that surgeon educators currently face is that attending surgeons have trouble identifying how much help they offer when assisting surgeon trainees, as discussed earlier.[27] The Zwisch scale associated with the SIMPL app used by multiple surgery programs to assess operative independence also takes this principle into account as it deciphers passive help versus supervision only.

### Educational Factors

When discussing potential barriers to resident autonomy, certainly behaviors and habits of faculty and residents play a role. Some of these factors overlap with issues discussed here regarding the importance of autonomy. For example, a resident who displays low levels of confidence or lack of patient ownership is likely to experience less autonomy. Other factors in the educational environment that are perceived barriers are discussed here.

In general, residents seem to believe they need more autonomy than faculty do; however, they both believe it to be important.[17] Faculty and residents also have trouble identifying the so-called magic hand or accurately assessing how much guidance is being offered by faculty assisting trainees.[27,28] These are seemingly modifiable but it is noteworthy that 2 studies have found that the greatest predictors of autonomy allowed to trainees are (1) trainee performance followed by (2) normally allowed autonomy by the attending or attending confidence.[10,55] This situation creates a significant barrier to autonomy for more complex operations and trainees who may be struggling compared with their peers.

Another barrier to autonomy has come to light largely through the efforts of the Procedural Learning and Safety Collaborative using the Zwisch scale for evaluation of operative autonomy using the SIMPL app across multiple institutions. Meyerson and colleagues[56] found that female surgery trainees are afforded less autonomy than their male counterparts in the largest and most recent study to date on operative autonomy in general surgery residents. Reasons for this disparity hypothesized by the investigators include gender-normative stereotypes as well as gender norms. They conclude that more research is required to better understand the impact of gender bias on surgery residents and surgery programs need to seek solutions.

## HOW CAN AUTONOMY IN GENERAL SURGERY TRAINING BE SUPPORTED?

The logical place to start with any discussion in support of autonomy is to address the barriers. Work has been done studying the effectiveness of patient education efforts with regard to improving patient receptiveness to resident involvement and resident autonomy.[37,39,40] These efforts are effective but they also show that the earlier resident involvement is introduced to patients, the more receptive patients are.[14,57] In addition, most of this work has been done using an educational intervention before the patients have even met their surgeons. Patients seem to assent more after they have been able to discuss involvement of trainees with their surgeons.[42,50] Attending surgeons can support resident autonomy merely by engaging in a conversation with their patients as early as possible about resident involvement as a matter of routine. In addition, the American College of Surgeons has created an informational pamphlet for the purpose of educating patients, entitled "What Is a Surgical Resident?" to assist in this effort.[58]

Residents who show a strong sense of patient ownership are also likely afforded more autonomy. The best method for faculty to support resident ownership of patients may be to solicit resident input when deciding to operate before weighing in on the decision themselves.[9,31] This method is also likely beneficial for developing confidence.[31] Further work to identify causes and solutions to gender gaps in autonomy afforded to residents is also needed.

Faculty development surrounding best practices in teaching is also likely valuable. Sandhu and colleagues[26] performed semistructured interviews of faculty and residents and identified 6 themes important to operative autonomy: optimize intraoperative feedback, regulations affecting resident participation, flexible faculty teaching strategies, resident preparedness and ownership, case leadership opportunities for the resident, and safe struggle when appropriate. Previous work has shown that often residents and faculty perceive learning needs differently, potentially hampering optimal learning.[28,59] Feedback alone is likely not enough for optimal learning, especially in those residents who may be struggling. Kruger and Dunning[36] state it well in their discussion, "The problem with failure is that it is subject to more attributional ambiguity than success [is]... Because of this, even if people receive feedback that points to a lack of skill, they may attribute it to some other factor." This statement highlights the importance of the attending surgeon as an active teacher and supervisor to produce well-trained general surgeons. The literature suggests that optimal learning occurs when the appropriate amount of safe struggle is allowed before takeover for the purpose of demonstrating best practices. Autonomy is also not an all-or-none phenomenon.

Many of the current evaluation tools (eg, the Zwisch scale) measure autonomy for the whole procedure but, in reality, residents are afforded autonomy earlier during certain portions of an operation and later as complexity increases. Ebeling and colleagues[60] showed that, in robot inguinal hernia repair, competency and autonomy increased faster during easier portions of the operation (eg, peritoneal flap closure) compared with more technically demanding portions (eg, hernia reduction). Extending autonomy during appropriate segments of surgical procedures or clinical encounters may lead to better learning and the best patient care. Further examination is warranted.

## SUMMARY

Lewis and Klingensmith[5] point out in their article delineating issues in general surgery training that it is "illogical and fallacious" to think that general surgery residents are completely ready for independent practice on the day of graduation but that 1 day before they are not, and they depend on attending supervision. Autonomy is critical to the training of independent practicing general surgeons. Much has been learned in the last 20 years about the need for and the effect of autonomy. The need for supervision has also been better delineated with benefit shown for the patient and trainee. Finding the optimal balance of trainee autonomy and attending supervision will allow the general surgery community to create the best clinical and educational outcomes into the future.

## DISCLOSURE

The authors report no proprietary or commercial interest in any product mentioned or concept discussed in this article.

## REFERENCES

1. Greene FL. Transition to practice: a bold move. Gen Surg News 2013;40(3):1.
2. Napolitano LM, Savarise M, Paramo JC, et al. Are general surgery residents ready to practice? A survey of the American College of Surgeons board of governors and Young Fellows Association. J Am Coll Surg 2014;218(5):1063–72.
3. Mattar SG, Alseidi AA, Jones DB, et al. General surgery residency inadequately prepares trainees for fellowship. Ann Surg 2013;258(3):440–9.
4. American College of Surgeons. Transition to practice program in general surgery: American College of Surgeons; Division of education. Available at: http://www.facs.org/ttp/index. Accessed November 19, 2020.
5. Lewis FR, Klingensmith ME. Issues in general surgery residency training–2012. Ann Surg 2012;256(4):553–9.
6. Bucholz EM, Sue GR, Yeo H, et al. Our trainees' confidence: results from a National Survey of 4136 US General Surgery Residents. Arch Surg 2011;146(8):907–14.
7. Bell RH. Why Johnny cannot operate. Surgery 2009;146(4):533–42.
8. Griner D, Menon RP, Kotwall CA, et al. The eighty-hour workweek: surgical attendings' perspectives. J Surg Educ 2010;67(1):25–31.
9. Randle RW, Ahle SL, Elfenbein DM, et al. Surgical trainees' sense of responsibility for patient outcomes: a multi-institutional appraisal. J Surg Res 2020;255:58–65.

10. Teman NR, Gauger PG, Mullan PB, et al. Entrustment of general surgery residents in the operating room: factors contributing to provision of resident autonomy. J Am Coll Surg 2014;219(4):778–87.
11. Santry HP, Chokski N, Datrice N, et al. General surgery training and the demise of the general surgeon. Bull Am Coll Surg 2008;93(7):32–8.
12. Chalabian J, Bremner R. The effects of programmatic change on resident motivation. Surgery 1998;123(5):511–7.
13. Babbott S. Commentary: watching closely at a distance: key tensions in supervising resident physicians. Acad Med 2010;85(9):1399–400.
14. Beale KG, Kempenich JW, Willis RE, et al. Surgical inpatient's attitudes toward resident participation: all about expectations. J Surg Educ 2020;77(6):e28–33.
15. Arriaga AF, Elbardissi AW, Regenbogen SE, et al. A policy-based intervention for the reduction of communication breakdowns in inpatient surgical care: results from Harvard surgical safety collaborative. Ann Surg 2011;253(5):849–54.
16. Asch DA, Parker RM. The Libby Zion case. One step forward or two steps backward. N Engl J Med 1988;318(12):771–5.
17. Kempenich JW, Willis RE, Rakosi R, et al. How do perceptions of autonomy differ in general surgery training between faculty, senior residents, hospital administrators, and the general public? A multi-institutional study. J Surg Educ 2015;72(6):e193–201.
18. Wong M, Gardiner E, Lang W, et al. Generational differences in personality and motivation: do they exist and what are the implications for the workplace? J Manag Psychol 2008;23(8):878–90.
19. Sterkenburg A, Barach P, Kalkman C, et al. When do supervising physicians decide to entrust residents with unsupervised tasks? Acad Med 2010;85(9):1408–17.
20. Bismuth H. Surgical specialization. Br J Surg 2013;100(S6):S43–4.
21. Doherty GM. Call to action for general surgery-trained specialists maintain both breadth and depth. JAMA Surg 2016;151(3):209–10.
22. Sachdeva AK, Bell RH, Britt LD, et al. National efforts to reform residency education in surgery. Acad Med 2007;82(12):1200–10.
23. ACGME program requirements for graduate medical education in general surgery. 2020. Available at: https://www.acgme.org/Portals/0/PFAssets/ProgramRequirements/440_GeneralSurgery_2020.pdf?ver=2020-06-22-085958-260.
24. Kusurkar R, tenCate O. AM last page: education is not filling a bucket, but lighting a fire: self-determination theory and motivation in medical students. Acad Med 2013;88(6):904.
25. Willis RE, Erwin D, Adelaja F. Struggling prior to a teaching even results in superior short-term skills acquisition in novice learners. J Surg Educ 2020;77(1):34–9.
26. Sandhu G, Magas CP, Robinson AB, et al. Progressive entrustment to achieve resident autonomy in the operating room. Ann Surg 2017;265(6):1134–40.
27. Chen X, Williams RG, Sanfey HA, et al. How do supervising surgeons evaluate guidance provided in the operating room? Am J Surg 2012;203(1):44–8.
28. Chen X, Williams RG, Smink DS. Do residents receive the same or guidance as surgeons report? Difference between residents' and surgeons' perceptions of OR guidance. J Surg Educ 2014;71(6):e79–82.
29. ABS E-News - Spring 2018: American Board of Surgery. 2018. Available at: https://www.absurgery.org/quicklink/absnews/absupdate0518.html. Accessed November 23, 2020.
30. Hinchey KT, Iwata I, Picchioni M, et al. "I can do patient care on my own": autonomy and the manager role. Acad Med 2009;84(11):1516–21.

31. Binenbaum G, Musick DW, Ross HM. The development of physician confidence during surgical and medical internship. Am J Surg 2007;193(1):79–85.

32. Wiggins-Dohlvik K, Stewart RM, Babbitt RJ, et al. Surgeons' performance during critical situations: competence, confidence, and composure. Am J Surg 2009; 198(6):817–23.

33. Cate Ot. Trust, competence, and the supervisor's role in postgraduate training. Br Med J 2006;333(7571):748–51.

34. Leopold SS, Morgan HD, Kadel NJ, et al. Impact of educational intervention on confidence and competence in the performance of a simple surgical task. J Bone Joint Surg Am 2005;87-A(5):1031–7.

35. Hassett JM, Zinnerstrom K, Nawotniak RH, et al. Utilization of standardized patients to evaluate clinical and interpersonal skills of surgical residents. Surgery 2006;140(4):633–9.

36. Kruger J, Dunning D. Unskilled and unaware of it: how difficulties in recognizing one's own incompetence lead to inflated self- assessments. J Pers Soc Psychol 1999;77(6):1121–34.

37. Kempenich JW, Willis RE, Blue RJ, et al. The effect of patient education on the perceptions of resident participation in surgical care. J Surg Educ 2016;73(6): e111–7.

38. O'Malley PG, Omori DM, Landry FJ, et al. A prospective study to assess the effect of ambulatory teaching on patient satisfaction. Acad Med 1997;72(11):1015–7.

39. Dickinson KJ, Bass BL, Nguyen DT, et al. Public perceptions of general surgery resident autonomy and supervision. J Am Coll Surg 2021;232(1):8–15.e1.

40. Kempenich JW, Willis RE, Fayyadh MA, et al. Video-based patient education improves patient attitudes toward resident participation in outpatient surgical care. J Surg Educ 2018;75(6):e61–7.

41. Cowles RA, Moyer CA, Sonnad SS, et al. Doctor-patient communication in surgery: attitudes and expectations of general surgery patients about the involvement and education of surgical residents. J Am Coll Surg 2001;193(1):73–80.

42. Petravick ME, Eddington JP, Idowu OA, et al. It all depends on who does what: a survey of patient and family member comfort with surgical trainees operating. J Surg Educ 2017;74(6):1001–6.

43. Scarborough JE, Bennett KM, Pappas TN. Defining the impact of resident participation on outcomes after appendectomy. Ann Surg 2012;255(3):577–82.

44. Iannuzzi JC, Chandra A, Rickles AS, et al. Resident involvement is associated with worse outcomes after major lower extremity amputation. J Vasc Surg 2013;58(3):827–31.

45. Davis SS, Husain FA, Lin E, et al. Resident participation in index laparoscopic general surgical cases: impact of the learning environment on surgical outcomes. J Am Coll Surg 2013;216(1):96–104.

46. Hernandez-Irizarry R, Zendejas B, Ali SM, et al. Impact of resident participation on laparoscopic inguinal hernia repairs: are residents slowing us down? J Surg Educ 2012;69(6):746–52.

47. Bakaeen FG, Dhaliwal AS, Chu D, et al. Does the level of experience of residents affect outcomes of coronary artery bypass surgery? Ann Thorac Surg 2009;87(4): 1127–33.

48. Hutter MM, Glasgow RE, Mulvihill SJ. Does the participation of a surgical trainee adversely impact patient outcomes? A study of major pancreatic resections in California. Surgery 2000;128(2):286–92.

49. Castleberry AW, Clary BM, Migaly J, et al. Resident education in the era of patient safety: a nationwide analysis of outcomes and complication in resident-assisted oncologic surgery. Ann Surg Oncol 2013;20:3715–24.
50. Counihan TC, Nye D, Wu JJ. Surgeons' experience with patients' concerns regarding trainees. J Surg Educ 2015;72(5):974–8.
51. Kairys JC, McGuire K, Crawford AG, et al. Cumulative operative experience is decreasing during general surgery residency: a worrisome trend for surgical trainees? J Am Coll Surg 2008;206(5):804–13.
52. Farnan JM, Petty LA, Georgitis E, et al. A systemic review: the effect of clinical supervision on patient and residency education outcomes. Grad Med Educ 2012;87(4):428–42.
53. Shetty K, Poo SXW, Sriskandarajah K, et al. "The longest way round is the shortest way home": an overhaul of surgical ward rounds. World J Surg 2018;42(4): 937–49.
54. Schmidt HG, Norman GR, Boshuizen HPA. A cognitive perspective on medical expertise: theory and implications. Acad Med 1990;65(10):611–21.
55. Williams RG, George BC, Meyerson SL, et al. What factors influence attending surgeon decisions about resident autonomy in the operating room? Surgery 2017;162(6):1314–9.
56. Meyerson SL, Odell DD, Zwischenberger JB, et al. The effect of gender on operative autonomy in general surgery residents. Surgery 2019;166(5):738–43.
57. Reichgott MJ, Schwartz JS. Acceptance by private patients of resident involvement in their outpatient care. J Med Educ 1983;58(9):703–9.
58. Copeland AW, Daly JM, Divino CM, et al. What is a surgical resident?: American College of Surgeons. Available at: https://www.facs.org/Education/Patient-Education/Patient-Resources/Prepare/Operation-and-Recovery/surgical-resident. Accessed November 24, 2020.
59. Pugh CM, DaRosa DA, Glenn D, et al. A comparison of faculty and resident perception of resident learning needs in the operating room. J Surg Educ 2007;64(5):250–5.
60. Ebeling PA, Beale KG, VanSickle KR, et al. Resident training experience with robotic assisted transabdominal preperitoneal inguinal hernia repair. Am J Surg 2020;219(2):278–82.

# Early Detection and Remediation of Problem Learners

Lilah F. Morris-Wiseman, MD, Valentine N. Nfonsam, MD, MS*

## KEYWORDS

- Remediation • Struggling learner • Surgical resident education

## KEY POINTS

- Most struggling surgical residents have difficulty in more than 1 competency area.
- Early identification of problem learners can be achieved by establishing a standard, objective curriculum of training and assessment.
- Once struggling learners are identified, the program team should identify a course of corrective action with clear delineation of the problem, methods for improvement, anticipated results, and consequences if remediation is not successful.

## INTRODUCTION

Residency program directors (PDs) serve as the gatekeepers for ensuring physicians are competent to enter practice.[1] Because of the high individual, programmatic, and societal investment in medical education, programs use performance improvement strategies for struggling residents that may include coaching and/or remediation.[2] The proportion of surgical residents who require remediation is highly variable and depends on both the individual program's assessment of acceptable performance and the degree of structured learning. Programs that focus more on structured, rather than experiential, learning may identify resident weaknesses that can be remedied by coaching with few residents requiring formal remediation.

## DEFINING A PROBLEM LEARNER

Struggling learners constitute a small proportion of surgical residents; 2% to 31% require remediation.[3–7] However, they represent a multifactorial problem that requires substantial time and monetary investment from the PD, faculty, and other residents.[8]

University of Arizona, Department of Surgery, Division of Surgical Oncology, 1501 N. Campbell Avenue, PO Box 245058, Tucson, AZ 85724-5058, USA
* Corresponding author.
*E-mail address:* vnfonsam@email.arizona.edu
Twitter: @valnfonsam (V.N.N.)

Surg Clin N Am 101 (2021) 611–624
https://doi.org/10.1016/j.suc.2021.05.008
0039-6109/21/© 2021 Elsevier Inc. All rights reserved.
surgical.theclinics.com

The American Board of Internal Medicine defined a problem resident as a trainee who shows a significant enough problem that requires intervention by someone of authority.[9] More specifically, a problem surgical resident is one who fails to meet expectations on 1 or more of the Accreditation Council on Graduate Medical Education (ACGME) core competencies.[10]

In general, surgical residents are not used to struggling or failure. They may be reluctant to believe there is a problem, blame others for the areas of concern, or attempt to avoid addressing deficiencies. Early identification and defining a clear problem and a path to remedy when residents do not meet performance criteria are essential.

Essential components of a remediation program for medical learners should (1) define acceptable performance criteria; (2) identify deficiencies via assessment using multiple valid, reliable tools or sources; (3) develop an individualized learning plan that clearly defines reassessment and metrics for success; (4) provide opportunities for deliberate practice, individualized coaching, timely feedback, and self-reflection; and (5) reassess for achievement of remediation goals and conclude remediation or initiate consequences for failure.[11,12]

## TYPES OF PROBLEM LEARNERS

Most problem residents have more than 1 area of deficiency in the realms of academic performance, clinical performance (applied knowledge or skills), and professional behavior.[4,6,13] The most common reason for resident remediation is deficiency in medical knowledge, followed by interpersonal and communication skills, and patient care (including poor clinical judgment or ineffective time management).[5,9] However, the most challenging resident problems may be behavioral, including poor relationships with health care team members.[13] The broad types of problem learners are outlined next.

### Does not meet objective knowledge expectations

As indicated, the most common resident problem requiring remediation–knowledge deficit–may present as faculty-reported low baseline knowledge or inability to grasp concepts quickly.[5,9] Interestingly, objective knowledge assessment via performance on the American Board of Surgery (ABS) In-Training Examination (ABSITE) has almost no association with faculty evaluation of resident performance.[14–16] Most general surgery PDs use 30th percentile as a passing ABSITE score because of data suggesting that examination performance below that level any time during residency was associated with failing the ABS Qualifying Examination (QE), and ABSITE score less than the 25th percentile predicted failure of both the QE and Certifying Examination (CE).[17,18]

Faculty evaluate technical skills subjectively in the patient care milestones 2 and 3 and objectively through the Fundamentals of Laparoscopic Skills (FLS) and Fundamentals of Endoscopic Skills (FES) examinations. The American College of Surgeons (ACS) and the Association of Program Directors in Surgery (APDS) developed a skills curriculum that includes a verification of proficiency (VOP) of the basic skills essential for junior residents, including knot tying; suturing; and insertion of central lines, chest drains, and emergency airways. Although this standardized method may identify problem learners early, it has not been widely used; more than half of surgery PDs do not think basic skills assessment is important for junior residents.[19] The Objective Structured Assessment of Technical Skills (OSATS), an assessment tool for grading technical proficiency in surgery, may also be able to discern struggling technical learners during their early residency.[20]

### Does not meet subjective evaluation expectations

Most residents struggle in more than 1 problem area, and combinations of problems may be difficult to navigate. For instance, Bergen and colleagues[21] defined problem residents with "synthetic defects" as "residents with an adequate knowledge base but difficulty interpreting and acting appropriately to clinical information." Of their 24 problem residents identified over a decade, all 4 of the residents who left the program involuntarily had synthetic defects as one of the multiple problem areas.[21] Residents with challenging interpersonal communication styles, lack of insight, and mental health disorders may be less likely to successfully complete remediation.[22]

Subjective assessment of learners relies on faculty feedback via rotation evaluations or operative performance assessments. Although the ACGME Core Competencies for general surgery have evolved to provide specific examples to aid in assessment, most programs offer little faculty training to assess competencies accurately.[22] End-of-rotation faculty evaluations of residents are often divergent, unreliable in identifying struggling residents, and unlikely to be able to differentiate one resident from another.[14,15] Faculty are frequently reluctant to evaluate residents honestly in writing, which limits the PD's ability to provide formative feedback.[4,9,23] Because evaluations so rarely contain negative feedback, residents with an outlier evaluation or evaluations containing neutral or negative words were significantly associated with residents requiring remediation.[2,24]

Insufficient objective information (faculty not writing what they think) and inexperienced or overburdened faculty are two common factors impeding identification of a struggling resident.[22] There is a significant reciprocity effect in general surgery residency evaluations, whereby faculty who give residents higher ratings on rotations evaluations are also rated higher by residents.[23] Reasons faculty are reluctant to document deficiencies, and almost never provide a failing evaluation for a failing trainee, include thinking that they may not have had enough time with the resident (lack of confidence in their assessment); fear of resident retaliation or need for a long appeals process that calls their credibility into question; uncertainty about what to document; and perceived lack of available remediation options (the perception that it was their job to provide remediation).[4,22,23,25]

### Junior problem learner

Because the skills required for success as a junior versus senior resident vary, residents may begin to struggle at different times.[4,7,13] Faculty may have low expectations of a junior resident's technical skills; as such, junior residents may not be flagged as struggling even when their basic technical skills are poor.[19] Junior problem learners may struggle with aspects of patient care (time management, efficiency, and attention to detail), medical knowledge, and behavioral skills.

## SENIOR PROBLEM LEARNER

Residents who are efficient, detail-oriented, personable, able to follow instructions, and dedicated to their work and self-improvement thrive as junior residents. However, senior residents must be able to make decisions independently, lead a team, and prepare for and lead operations. Because of the hierarchical nature of surgical teams, residents who struggle with these complex issues may not be apparent to faculty until they reach the senior years, which can be challenging. Residents at postgraduate year (PGY) 3 or later have already invested several years into a program with seeming success as junior residents. Residents may begin to experience a spiral of failure as additional responsibility brings many deficiencies to light.[26] Struggling senior residents may try to limit exposure to areas of deficiency (eg, avoid challenging operative cases); they must be identified promptly and remediated with clear expectations for outcomes.

### Lack of insight

The highest-performing residents tend to underestimate their skills, whereas the lowest-performing residents tend to profoundly overestimate their competency-specific performance in behavioral skills such as interpersonal skills, communication, teamwork, and professionalism.[27] Interestingly, lack of insight is not a common reason for failure of remediation.[28] However, residents who have insight into their deficiencies and who are invested in the self-improvement process have the best chance of succeeding in remediation.[22]

### Early detection of the problem learner

#### Applicant Selection

Individualized, values-based program recruitment can decrease remediation and attrition in a surgical residency program.[29] Although programs must define and understand their own culture and values, applicant interviews that explore whether prospective residents have social support, strategies for time management, ability to work in teams, and strategies to manage failure may be able to better predict success.[30] However, using resident characteristics to predict problem learners may introduce bias. In 1 study, expert opinion identified international medical graduates (IMGs) and residents from underrepresented minority groups as those more likely to need remediation. However, as the percentage of residents from these groups increased within programs, PDs were less concerned about their potential for poor performance.[5,9,21,30] IMGs were significantly less likely to be identified as problem residents in programs with high proportions of IMG residents.[9] Thus, programs should recognize the potential for bias and avoid any residency selection criteria that associate specific, personal, or immutable resident characteristics with failure.

Professionalism lapses as medical students predict professionalism-related problems during residency. In a case-control study, medical students who had formal professionalism concerns (ie, had to appear before their school's review board) were 5 times more likely to undergo disciplinary review during residency (16% vs 3% respectively) and 4 times more likely to require remediation (35% vs 9%).[31] During the interview process, it is important to seek and weigh heavily input from residents and program administrative staff to ensure that behavior during the faculty interview is consistent with that shown to others.[30]

#### Objective Skills Assessment

Feedback and objective skills assessment on clinical rotations are challenging. Residents must have the opportunity to practice particular skills repetitively, and faculty must be trained in providing objective feedback and commit time to this activity. There are several published models that programs have used to internally and objectively critically assess residents' performance, including Mayo Clinic Rochester's Surgical X-Games and Harbor University of California, Los Angeles Medical Center's Surgical Trainee Assessment of Readiness.[32,33] These structured clinical examinations, like the OSATS and VOP, provide residents with detailed, specific, constructive, and relevant feedback to guide improvement and allow opportunities for retesting to obtain proficiency.[20,32–34] The use of expected remediation required in these models may normalize identification of deficiencies, coaching, and mentored practice.

*Faculty Feedback*

As discussed, faculty end-of-rotation evaluations may not be helpful in identifying problem learners.[2,22,24] Faculty are reluctant to detail resident concerns in written format, preferring private or verbal communication, because of fear of resident retaliation, lack of confidence in their assessments, and fear that nothing will change after reporting the behavior.[4,25,30] PDs can (and should) document verbal concerns expressed to them with regard to a resident's performance.

Faculty group evaluations may reveal a pattern of performance and provide an opportunity for individuals to discuss concerns that they may have been reluctant to voice otherwise.[25,35] Faculty who have been hesitant to fail a trainee for failing performance are more willing to honestly assess the trainee if others also thought the trainee's performance was failing.[36] Faculty discussions may identify deficient resident performance that was not documented on postrotation performance evaluation.[25,35]

*Early Resident Review (First 6 Months) Using Reliable Assessments*

ABSITE scores released at approximately 8 months after starting residency may delay early identification of problem learners. Administering an earlier standardized examination to residents and grading predidactic and postdidactic questions have been shown to predict in-training examination performance.[37,38]

Clinical competency committee (CCC) meetings are required by the ACGME only semiannually. Holding monthly CCC meetings to review 1 class at a time, discuss any resident concerns, and review progress for problem learners may be able to identify struggling residents early and provide an opportunity for rapid intervention.[39]

## PROGRAM-LEVEL ASSESSMENT AND REMEDIATION STRATEGIES
*Normalizing Feedback and Remediation: How to Avoid Labeling a Resident*

Routine and comprehensive assessment coupled with remediation when necessary is a critical component of any surgery residency program. The challenges of an elaborate assessment program are enormous; every residency PD can attest to this. In order to better help a struggling resident, an unbiased but unvarnished truthful evaluation is warranted. These evaluations include formal end-of-rotation evaluations from both faculty and senior residents and informal but appropriately documented discussions between the PD and any informal faculty evaluator. Dudek and colleagues[36] discussed the challenges faced by faculty in failing poorly performing residents. Grade inflation was common because faculty were unwilling to give poor evaluations because of fear of negative consequences to the faculty as well as the resident.[36]

Ideally, when a residency program establishes a culture of excellence, remediation can be part of a regular curricular program and nonpunitive.[40] Surgery residents who are used to excelling in academics may view negative evaluations as failure and respond with defensiveness and anger at the evaluator rather than receiving feedback as an opportunity for advancement.[26] Emphasizing that residents should learn and grow throughout the program and setting the expectation for progressive, competency-based feedback may assist with this process.

Described by Kalet and colleagues,[40] "Remediation should be reframed from a matter of punishment and stigma to a form of training that many, if not most, will need and benefit from at some point." To that end, every resident should be tasked with self-identifying or working with a mentor to identify their personal areas of weakness and opportunities for growth. To build a transparent process for feedback and remediation, residents should be encouraged to discuss these areas with faculty when beginning a rotation and request specific feedback related to that skill or competency. In this way, remediation becomes a part of natural educational development rather than a punishment.

## Types of Problem Learners and Best-practice Remediation Strategies for Individual Residents

In order to be effective, remediation must be systematic, targeted, and individualized with defined expectations and outcomes. Remediation cannot provide more of the same to learners like additional intensive teaching.[41] Successful remediation supports the development of tools for success in the form of effective lifelong learning skills and requires expertise from multiple specialists.[41,42] Remediation teams tasked with mentoring and coaching may consist of the PD or other surgical faculty, an education specialist, and a mental health professional.[6,42,43] Faculty competency champions can be used as experts in their particular competency to help remediate struggling residents and normalize remediation.[39] Given conflicting motivations, the remediation team should be separated from those deciding the outcome of remediation.[42,43] Despite these studied recommendations, most general surgery resident remediation programs are developed and monitored by the PD without a standard consequence of the inability to complete remediation.[11]

## Patient Care: Clinical Skills, Clinical Reasoning, Organization, and Time Management

### Skills-based assessment/remediation

The most common methods for remediating surgery residents are to increase direct observation by faculty of residents in clinic, operating room, and wards and provide more mentorship, feedback, and skills training.[7,11] Use of available, validated methods by which to assess clinical competency helps to show specific expectations, assess performance, and set future goals for optimal performance. The Clinical Assessment and Management Evaluation (CAMEO) includes a structure for faculty and patient feedback from an observed resident initial patient evaluation (https://www.absurgery.org/default.jsp?certgsqe_resassess). Entrustable professional activities (EPAs) are responsibilities that residents are expected to perform independently by the conclusion of training.[44] Rating systems for a particular EPA, such as management of right lower quadrant pain, are focused on the level of supervision required for preoperative, intraoperative, and postoperative performance. Because these evaluations relate to a particular event or patient, they may be completed rapidly with the goal of increasing the number of evaluations received per resident and detecting outliers in expected performance. Approximately 40% of plastic surgery residency programs use objective structured clinical examinations (OSCEs) to assess all of the milestone categories.[45]

### Operating room assessment/remediation

There are several key aspects of operative performance: technical skills (use surgical instruments efficiently and effectively), forward planning (anticipate needs and set up the operation optimally), self-direction (conduct oneself professionally, stay focused, slow down when appropriate, and accept and respond to feedback), patient safety and judgment (intraoperative decision making), and situational awareness (assess and interpret cues from the environment and provide team leadership).[46,47] To form a valuable and more objective assessment tool, operative evaluations need to be completed more frequently (at least 20 per year) by multiple observers.[46,48] The briefing, intraoperative teaching, and debriefing model may be used for directed rather than exploratory learning.[49,50] There remains no standard for operative teaching, what constitutes mastery, and what level of proficiency or autonomy is required for graduating residents.[49] Although case logs are required for certification, it is the PD who is responsible for certifying the resident's operative performance.

Minter and colleagues[47] propose specific steps to identify deficiencies in operative skills with correlative remedies. Allowing the resident autonomy in leading the operation may uncover poor forward planning or deficiencies in patient safety and judgment. These deficiencies may be remedied by asking the resident to design a preoperative "flight plan" or rehearsal of steps. Poor situational awareness includes not recognizing needed equipment, patient positioning, antibiotics, or anesthetic concerns. There are multiple checklist-type systems available that can assist with remedying this deficiency.[47]

## Medical Knowledge

### American Board of Surgery In-Training Examination
The ABSITE is used to test residents' cumulative knowledge, prepare residents for the QE and CE, and assist residency programs in evaluating the effectiveness of their academic programs. A recent meta-analysis showed that the most effective remediation programs to improve individual ABSITE scores are mandatory, multimodal programs and ones that use e-learning (learning management systems, an online software platform that automates the administration, tracking, and reporting of training) and social media.[51–53] One study found a 3 percentage point increase in ABSITE score for every 100 practice questions completed.[54] Increased use of the Surgical Council on Resident Education (SCORE) curriculum (measured by total minutes and total visits) has been associated with an increase in ABSITE percentile scores and in first-time QE and CE board pass rates.[53] Programs that track resident reading have higher median ABSITE scores than programs that do not.[55]

### Medical knowledge in practice
Many struggling learners who describe that they do not "test well" lack the appropriate systems to study efficiently and effectively in a fast-paced and dynamic environment. Struggling learners must understand that their deficits are not part of their innate ability. They may have poor knowledge of task requirements, lack recognition of their own level of expertise, and have problematic self-regulatory skills such as ineffective learning strategies and maladaptive motivational beliefs. Self-Regulated Learning–Microanalytic Assessment and Training is an assessment framework to address these deficits.[56] Struggling learners can be taught to improve their performance by learning to set goals, develop strategic plans, self-monitor, and evaluate their own performance.

Clinical judgment is a broad area that may be best assessed and remediation approached based on the type of deficiency. Minter and colleagues[47] described sources of poor judgment. An overconfident so-called cowboy resident who resists supervision should be told there is a zero-tolerance policy for such unprofessional behavior and failure to communicate. A minimizer resident may underemphasize important clinical issues and must be counseled to provide clear, objective data rather than a potentially overly optimistic interpretation. A worrier may keep patients in the hospital longer, order more testing, and always be searching for potential complications. This resident should be counseled to trust objective data to make decisions. Residents who are able to create a common differential diagnosis list but do not consider worst-case diagnoses must be challenged in repeated clinical settings by different attendings to consider all possible scenarios so as to not miss anything. Residents who inappropriately defer to faculty preference rather than formulating their own plans need to be pushed to create their own plans, with faculty working to positively reinforce any reasonable plan.[47]

### Professionalism

The ACGME Surgery Core Competency for Professionalism encompasses use of ethical principles in patient care decision making, professional behavior and decision making (setting limits, performs responsibilities in a timely manner, and takes responsibility for behavior), completion of administrative tasks in a timely manner, and self-awareness and help seeking. Professionalism deficiencies are serious and sometimes difficult to remediate.[6]

The first phase of many professionalism interventions involves identifying the problem through feedback from multiple sources to bring awareness to the issue or psychometric testing.[57,58] Most interventions involve behavior change techniques and use individualized learning plans with didactic methods, small group learning, simulation and role play, or a coaching model, followed by reflection; punitive consequences (probation status or requirement to attend remediation); and structured mentoring by senior resident or faculty surgeon.[30,57] Failure to enforce consequences of poor professional performance can negatively affect behavior and morale of other residents and the health system as a whole.[30,59] Academic deficiencies must be differentiated from misconduct: behavior that is wrong and that the person knows is wrong will not be remedied with remediation.[30]

### Systems-based Practice

The systems-based practice milestone assesses the resident's knowledge and practice of patient safety and quality improvement, care coordination, and optimizing practice delivery systems. Residents who do not meet these milestones can be coached through undergoing individual faculty tutoring, being paired with senior residents for remediation, leading a multidisciplinary case conference, completing a quality improvement project, and giving a presentation on cost-effective health care.[58] This work is often completed outside of faculty observation but may be observed objectively through an OSCE.[45]

### Practice-based Learning and Improvement

Often evaluated with systems-based practice, practice-based learning and improvement requires learners to use evidence to inform their surgical practice and commit to personal growth. Assessment of this milestone is often subjective, involving reviewing resident portfolios or a general impression of whether the resident is committed to improvement.[60] Ways to remediate deficiencies in this milestone include assigning the resident to lead a journal club, improve existing conferences, and work with a faculty mentor to critically appraise scientific literature.[58] However, few remediation programs discuss this milestone, and many programs do not think that specific remediation in this area has been necessary.[58]

### Interpersonal and Communication Skills

Although tied with professionalism, communication skills milestones are focused on resident communication with patients, interprofessional teams, and within health systems (eg, communication within the medical record). Poor communication is a cause of about 20% of surgeon malpractice claims and is common among surgeons in practice who struggle to pass the ABS CE.[11,61] Communication skills can be assessed through direct observation of patient encounters, OSCE with a standardized patient, and 360° peer, nursing, or patient evaluations.[45,62]

Learners can remediate communication skills by watching and reflecting on their own performance in clinical settings, direct coaching with a standardized patient, role play, and structured feedback.[62] Asking residents to focus on and model excellent peer behavior can create a coaching relationship between junior and senior residents. Although not designed for remediation, programs that give residents tools to improve emotional intelligence, empathy, and reactivity may also improve communication.[63]

## WHEN AND HOW TO INTERVENE?

Although many struggling residents have difficulty in more than 1 domain, focusing remediation efforts in a stepwise fashion that allows for success in 1 area before moving to the next is critical. Someone should intervene with a struggling resident as soon as a deficiency is identified by implementing a performance improvement plan within which reevaluation is incorporated.

### How to Write a Performance Improvement Plan

The PD should document formally a deficiency and necessary steps toward improvement. Recent efforts have attempted to standardize the terminology of remediation with clear phases progressing from coaching and informal remediation (warning stage with letter of concern, corrective action plan, or professional development plan, with only program-level involvement), to formal remediation (involving Graduate Medical Education [GME] office at an institutional level), to probation, and concluding with termination if all other efforts are unsuccessful. Essential elements of such a document include a clear, evidence-based statement of the issues, a detailed action plan with measurable outcomes and timeline for completion, a clear statement of the consequences for not remediating, a reference to the due process at the institution, and acknowledgment that evaluations are based on expert opinions of educators (standard remediation contracts are available from Moffett and colleagues[64]).

## CHALLENGES IN REMEDIATION

One of the challenges of remediation in residency lies in institutions with less educational flexibility where moving a resident to a different rotation or taking a resident off service completely in order to focus on educational remediation creates a gap in the workflow.[40] Although discussed elsewhere, other challenges in remediation arise when there is a wide variability in subjective assessments or variation between objective results and subjective assessments (eg, excellent ABSITE scores in a resident who behaves unprofessionally). Gender or racial bias is inherent in subjective assessments. Systemic bias in medicine limits success of groups traditionally underrepresented in surgery.

## NOT ALL CAN BE REMEDIATED: SUCCESS OF REMEDIATION AND ATTRITION

Competing interests are involved in remediation of struggling resident learners. In surgical residency, learners may have large undergraduate and medical school debts and may not be able to obtain another comparable position without completing the program. There are societal implications related to patient safety and appropriate use of testing/systems in physicians who lack appropriate patient care skills. There is a major faculty time investment in struggling learners.

Despite the residency program's duty to train competent surgeons and protect the public from potential harm, most faculty do not fail failing trainees.[36] Barriers to failing trainees were lack of documentation, concern about an appeal that would call the evaluator's credibility into question, and a lack of known remediation options. A survey of general surgery PDs found that none would prevent residents with poor basic surgical skills from being promoted.[19]

Most residents successfully complete remediation and return to good academic standing and graduate.[3,6,13,21] Residents who are most successful with remediation are those with poor performance on in-training examination, inefficient time management, and inability to maintain proper medical records.[65] Poor professionalism has been a predictor of unsuccessful remediation, as has lack of engagement in remediation efforts or refusal to address the underlying problem (ie, mental health or medical condition).[6,28] Residents with challenging interpersonal communication styles, lack of insight, and mental health disorders may be less likely to successfully complete remediation.[22]

Yearly attrition from surgery residency is 2.4% and cumulative 5-year attrition rate is 12.9%.[66] Most residents (65%) who exit surgery residency do so in the first 2 years of training and most residents who leave surgical training enter another GME training program.[66,67] Termination, or involuntary attrition, is rare (0.4% of all trainees) and is most common in PGY3 and PGY4.[67]

Most studies define success of remediation as program graduation. However, long-term outcomes of struggling learners have not been well studied. Williams and colleagues[13] found that more than 40% of residents who required remediation did not have board certification in any specialty after an average of 11 years out of the program. Additional research that follows residents longitudinally to determine the impact of remediation is needed.

## SUMMARY

Early identification of struggling learners can be accomplished methodologically through objective assessment. Defining clear expectations, using objective methods to identify specific deficiencies, and providing feedback on achievement creates a culture of learning and self-improvement and avoids the stigma of remediation.

## DISCLOSURE

The authors have nothing to disclose.

## REFERENCES

1. Schenarts PJ, Langenfeld S. The fundamentals of resident dismissal. Am Surg 2017;83(2):119–26.

2. Rumack CM, Guerrasio J, Christensen A, et al. Academic remediation: why early identification and intervention matters. Acad Radiol 2017;24(6):730–3.

3. Schwed AC, Lee SL, Salcedo ES, et al. Association of general surgery resident remediation and program director attitudes with resident attrition. JAMA Surg 2017;152(12):1134–40.

4. Bhatti NI, Ahmed A, Stewart MG, et al. Remediation of problematic residents - A national survey. Laryngoscope 2016;126(4):834–8.

5. Yaghoubian A, Galante J, Kaji A, et al. General surgery resident remediation and attrition a multi-institutional study. Arch Surg 2012;147(9):829–33.

6. Guerrasio J, Garrity MJ, Aagaard EM. Learner deficits and academic outcomes of medical students, residents, fellows, and attending physicians referred to a remediation program, 2006-2012. Acad Med 2014;89(2):352–8.

7. Melton W, Jackson JB, Koon D, et al. Orthopaedic resident remediation. JBJS Open Access 2018;3(4):e0011.

8. Gardner AK, Grantcharov T, Dunkin BJ. The science of selection: using best practices from industry to improve success in surgery training. J Surg Educ 2018;75(2):278–85.

9. Yao DC, Wright SM. National survey of internal medicine residency program directors regarding problem residents. J Am Med Assoc 2000;284(9):1099–104.

10. The Accreditation Council for Graduate Medical Education. Surgery milestones 2019;Version 2(December 2013) Available at: https://www.acgme.org/Portals/0/PDFs/Milestones/SurgeryMilestones.pdf. Accessed January 2019.

11. Griffen FD. ACS Closed Claims Study reveals critical failures to communicate. Bull Am Coll Surg 2007;92(1):11–6.

12. Hauer KE, Ciccone A, Henzel TR, et al. Remediation of the deficiencies of physicians across the continuum from medical school to practice: a thematic review of the literature. Acad Med 2009;84(12):1822–32.

13. Williams RG, Roberts NK, Schwind CJ, et al. The nature of general surgery resident performance problems. Surgery 2009;145(6):651–8.

14. Ray JJ, Sznol JA, Teisch LF, et al. Association between American Board of Surgery In-Training Examination scores and resident performance. JAMA Surg 2016;151(1):26–31.

15. Elfenbein DM, Sippel RS, McDonald R, et al. Faculty evaluations of resident medical knowledge: can they be used to predict American Board of Surgery In-Training Examination performance? Am J Surg 2015;209(6):1095–101.

16. Kimbrough MK, Thrush CR, Barrett E, et al. Are surgical milestone assessments predictive of in-training examination scores? J Surg Educ 2018;75(1):29–32.

17. Taggarshe D, Mittal V. The utility of the ABS in-training examination (ABSITE) score forms: percent correct and percentile score in the assessment of surgical residents. J Surg Educ 2012;69(4):554–8.

18. de Virgilio C, Chan T, Kaji A, et al. Weekly assigned reading and examinations during residency, ABSITE Performance, and improved pass rates on the American Board of Surgery examinations. J Surg Educ 2008;65(6):499–503.

19. Sanfey HA, Dunnington GL. Basic surgical skills testing for junior residents: current views of general surgery program directors. J Am Coll Surg 2011;212(3):406–12.

20. de Montbrun S, Louridas M, Grantcharov T. Passing a technical skills examination in the first year of surgical residency can predict future performance. J Grad Med Educ 2017;9(3):324–9.

21. Bergen PC, Littlefield JH, O'keefe GE, et al. Identification of high-risk residents. J Surg Res 2000;92(2):239–44.

22. Krzyzaniak SM, Wolf SJ, Byyny R, et al. A qualitative study of medical educators' perspectives on remediation: Adopting a holistic approach to struggling residents. Med Teach 2017;39(9):967–74.

23. Gardner AK, Scott DJ. Repaying in kind: examination of the reciprocity effect in faculty and resident evaluations. J Surg Educ 2016;73(6):e91–4.

24. Guerrasio J, Cumbler E, Trosterman A, et al. Determining need for remediation through postrotation evaluations. J Grad Med Educ 2012;4(1):47–51.

25. Schwind CJ, Williams RG, Boehler ML, et al. Do individual attendings' post-rotation performance ratings detect residents' clinical performance deficiencies? Acad Med 2004;79(5):453–7.
26. McLeod K, Waller S, King D, et al. Struggling urology trainee: a qualitative study into causes of underperformance. ANZ J Surg 2020;90(6):991–6.
27. Lipsett PA, Harris I, Downing S. Resident self-other assessor agreement: influence of assessor, competency, and performance level. Arch Surg 2011; 146(8):901.
28. Guerrasio J, Brooks E, Rumack CM, et al. The evolution of resident remedial teaching at one institution. Acad Med 2019;94(12):1891–4.
29. Kelz RR, Mullen JL, Kaiser LR, et al. Prevention of surgical resident attrition by a novel selection strategy. Ann Surg 2010;252(3):537–41.
30. Sanfey H, Darosa DA, Hickson GB, et al. Pursuing professional accountability an evidence-based approach to addressing residents with behavioral problems. Arch Surg 2012;147(7):642–7.
31. Krupat E, Dienstag JL, Padrino SL, et al. Do professionalism lapses in medical school predict problems in residency and clinical practice? Acad Med 2020; 95(6):888–95.
32. Gas BL, Buckarma ELH, Mohan M, et al. Objective assessment of general surgery residents followed by remediation. J Surg Educ 2016;73(6):e71–6.
33. Dauphine C, Neville AL, Moazzez A, et al. Can deficiencies in performance be identified earlier in surgical residency? An initial report of a surgical trainee assessment of readiness exam. J Surg Educ 2018;75(6):e91–6.
34. Beason AM, Hitt CE, Ketchum J, et al. Verification of proficiency in basic skills for PGY-1 surgical residents: 10-year update. J Surg Educ 2019;76(6):e217–24.
35. Wu JS, Siewert B, Boiselle PM. Resident evaluation and remediation: a comprehensive approach. J Grad Med Educ 2010;2(2):242–5.
36. Dudek NL, Marks MB, Regehr G. Failure to fail: the perspectives of clinical supervisors. Acad Med 2005;80(10):S84–7.
37. Corneille MG, Willis R, Stewart RM, et al. Performance on brief practice examination identifies residents at risk for poor ABSITE and ABS qualifying examination performance. J Surg Educ 2011;68(3):246–9.
38. Platt MP, Davis EM, Grundfast K, et al. Early detection of factual knowledge deficiency and remediation in otolaryngology residency education. Laryngoscope 2014;124(8):E309–11.
39. Ketteler ER, Auyang ED, Beard KE, et al. Competency champions in the clinical competency committee: a successful strategy to implement milestone evaluations and competency coaching. J Surg Educ 2014;71(1):36–8.
40. Kalet A, Chou CL, Ellaway RH. To fail is human: remediating remediation in medical education. Perspect Med Educ 2017;6(6):418–24.
41. Cleland J, Leggett H, Sandars J, et al. The remediation challenge: theoretical and methodological insights from a systematic review. Med Educ 2013;47(3):242–51.
42. Chou CL, Kalet A, Costa MJ, et al. Guidelines: the dos, don'ts and don't knows of remediation in medical education. Perspect Med Educ 2019;8(6):322–38.
43. Kalet A, Guerrasio J, Chou CL. Twelve tips for developing and maintaining a remediation program in medical education. Med Teach 2016;38(8):787–92.
44. Steiman J, Sullivan SA, Scarborough J, et al. Measuring competence in surgical training through assessment of surgical entrustable professional activities. J Surg Educ 2018;75(6):1452–62.

45. Simmons BJ, Zoghbi Y, Askari M, et al. Significance of objective structured clinical examinations to plastic surgery residency training. Ann Plast Surg 2017; 79(3):312–9.
46. Sanfey H, Williams R, Dunnington G. Recognizing residents with a deficiency in operative performance as a step closer to effective remediation. J Am Coll Surg 2013;216(1):114–22.
47. Minter RM, Dunnington GL, Sudan R, et al. Can this resident be saved? Identification and early intervention for struggling residents. J Am Coll Surg 2014;219(5): 1088–95.
48. Williams RG, Verhulst S, Colliver JA, et al. A template for reliable assessment of resident operative performance: Assessment intervals, numbers of cases and raters. Surgery 2012;152(4):517–27.
49. Williams RG, George BC, Bohnen JD, et al. A proposed blueprint for operative performance training, assessment, and certification. Ann Surg 2020;273(4): 701–8.
50. Roberts NK, Williams RG, Kim MJ, et al. The briefing, intraoperative teaching, debriefing model for teaching in the operating room. J Am Coll Surg 2009;208(2): 299–303.
51. Decoteau MA, Rivera L, Umali K, et al. A multimodal approach improves American Board of Surgery In-Training Examination scores. Am J Surg 2018;215(2): 315–21.
52. Cheun TJ, Davies MG. Improving ABSITE scores - a meta-analysis of reported remediation models. Am J Surg 2020;220(6):1557–65.
53. Williams TP, Hancock KJ, Klimberg S, et al. Learning to read: successful program-based remediation using the Surgical Council on Resident Education (SCORE) curriculum. J Am Coll Surg 2021;232(4):397–403.
54. Flentje AO, Caturegli I, Kavic SM. Practice makes perfect: introducing a question bank for ABSITE preparation improves program performance. J Surg Educ 2020; 77(1):54–60.
55. Kim JJ, Gifford ED, Moazzez A, et al. Program factors that influence American Board of Surgery In-Training Examination Performance: a multi-institutional study. J Surg Educ 2015;72(6):e236–42.
56. Durning SJ, Cleary TJ, Sandars J, et al. Perspective: viewing "strugglers" through a different lens: how a self-regulated learning perspective can help medical educators with assessment and remediation. Acad Med 2011;86(4):488–95.
57. Brennan N, Price T, Archer J, et al. Remediating professionalism lapses in medical students and doctors: a systematic review. Med Educ 2020;54(3):196–204.
58. Torbeck L, Canal DF. Remediation practices for surgery residents. Am J Surg 2009;197(3):397–402.
59. Hickson GB, Pichert JW, Webb LE, et al. A complementary approach to promoting professionalism: identifying, measuring, and addressing unprofessional behaviors. Acad Med 2018;82(11):1040–8.
60. Wu BJ, Dietz PA, Bordley IVJ, et al. A novel, web-based application for assessing and enhancing practice-based learning in surgery residency. J Surg Educ 2009; 66(1):3–7.
61. Rowland PA, Trus TL, Lang NP, et al. The certifying examination of the American Board of Surgery: the effect of improving communication and professional competency: Twenty-year results. J Surg Educ 2012;69(1):118–25.
62. Al-Sheikhly D, Östlundh L, Arayssi T. Remediation of learners struggling with communication skills: a systematic review. BMC Med Educ 2020;20(1):215.

63. Price ET, Coverley CR, Arrington AK, et al. Are we making an impact? A qualitative program assessment of the resident leadership, well-being, and resiliency program for general surgery residents. J Surg Educ 2020;77(3):508–19.

64. Moffett P, Lefebvre C, Williamson K. Standardized letters of concern and remediation contracts: templates for program directors. J Grad Med Educ 2019;11(5): 606–10.

65. Badran KW, Kelley K, Conderman C, et al. Improving applicant selection: Identifying qualities of the unsuccessful otolaryngology resident. Laryngoscope 2015; 125(4):842–7.

66. Shweikeh F, Schwed AC, Hsu CH, et al. Status of resident attrition from surgical residency in the past, present, and future outlook. J Surg Educ 2018;75(2): 254–62.

67. Yeo H, Bucholz E, Sosa JA, et al. A national study of attrition in general surgery training: Which residents leave and where do they go? Ann Surg 2010;252(3): 529–34.

# Maintaining Wellness and Instilling Resilience in General Surgeons

Jessica Brittany Weiss, MD, Michael Minh Vu, MD,
Quinton Morrow Hatch, MD, Vance Young Sohn, MD*

## KEYWORDS

• Wellness • Resilience • Burnout

## KEY POINTS

• Fostering wellness occurs through a deliberate series of conscious actions that leads to increased resilience and career satisfaction.
• Resiliency can be taught and refined.
• Wellness and resilience are interconnected and must be emphasized during training as a step in turning the tide of surgeon burnout.

The concept of wellness is not new, having its roots in ancient civilizations. However, the modern view of wellness has evolved over just the last half century with increasing interest and research beginning in the 1970s. Over this same time period, there have been significant changes in medical practice and an evolving focus on wellness in surgical education. However, despite increased focus on wellness and reforms in surgical education, the level of burnout and career dissatisfaction is at an all-time high with rates of suicide and depression among physicians outpacing the general public.[1–3] This review provides an overview of the current landscape from the perspective of wellness and explores measures that can be taken to improve resiliency to protect against burnout.

## THE ORIGINS OF MODERN WELLNESS

The idea of wellness has its foundations in ancient societies including Ayurvedic practices in India and traditional Chinese medicine. These cultures emphasized connection and harmony between the mind, body, and spirit as the key to health. Ancient Greek medicine also acknowledged that health goes beyond simply treating illness and

Department of Surgery, Madigan Army Medical Center, 9040 Fitzsimmons Drive, Joint Base Lewis McChord, WA 98433, USA
* Corresponding author.
E-mail address: vance.y.sohn.mil@mail.mil

Surg Clin N Am 101 (2021) 625–634
https://doi.org/10.1016/j.suc.2021.05.009
0039-6109/21/Published by Elsevier Inc.

recognized the importance of disease prevention through lifestyle modification to overall health.[4]

The concept of wellness regained attention in modern medicine after World War II with the founding of the World Health Organization (WHO) in 1948. In the preamble to its constitution, the WHO defines health as "a state of complete physical, mental and social wellbeing, and not merely the absence of disease and infirmity." Dr Halbert Dunn, a physician consultant to the WHO, was inspired by this concept of health and introduced the idea of wellness as a positive concept of health, rather than a simple absence of illness.[5] In his writings throughout the 1950s, Dunn worked to define levels of wellness and called on physicians and public health officials to assist in working toward this positive definition of health and the idea of high-level wellness.[6,7] This concept of wellness started to take hold in the United States in the 1970s when Dr John Travis, influenced by the writings of Dunn, opened the first wellness center, marking a period of increased interest in the concept of wellness that continues today.[4,5]

## DEFINING WELLNESS AND IDENTIFYING BURNOUT

Despite many publications on the subject since the 1970s, there remains no consensus definition of wellness. This is at least in part due to the relative and subjective nature of wellness. In his seminal writings on the subject, Dunn incorporated physical, mental, and social well-being at the individual, family, and society into his definition of high-level wellness. Despite this lack of consensus, it has become clear that self-perceived levels of wellness have been declining across all medical specialties, with surgeons and surgeons in training among the groups most affected.[2,8–10]

Burnout is a concept complementary to wellness that classically applies to professions in which human interaction is a central component, such as in medicine. Burnout is defined as a constellation of symptoms to include emotional exhaustion, depersonalization, and diminished satisfaction with work.[11] These features are quantified by the Maslach Burnout Inventory (MBI) and have been used across numerous studies to evaluate physician well-being. The MBI is a 22-item inventory that evaluates symptoms of burnout on 3 scales: emotional exhaustion, depersonalization, and personal accomplishment.[11]

Multiple studies have suggested that burnout has been increasing among physicians and trainees over the course of the twenty-first century.[1,2,10] Furthermore, surgeons and surgical residents have been identified as particularly at risk groups for burnout.[9,12,13] The high prevalence of burnout has consequences on both the personal and system level. At the individual level, burnout is associated with increased rates of depression, alcohol and substance misuse, and suicidality.[14,15] At the system level, increased burnout has been linked to worse patient outcomes, increased medical errors, and physician turnover.[1,16,17] These consequences have immense implications for the health care environment, including monetary effects, and they are being increasingly recognized in mainstream culture.[18] This attention has led to some changes in the landscape of medical and surgical training.

## THE EVOLUTION OF SURGICAL TRAINING AND ITS IMPACT ON WELLNESS

The death of Libby Zion in 1984, the daughter of a journalist and former lawyer, shed light on the culture of medical training and provoked a shift in the approach to physician training. The grand jury investigation into the death centered around excessive duty hours by resident physicians and the lack of supervision as the primary contributors to her death.[19,20] The grand jury proceedings ultimately led to the formation of a state committee to evaluate the condition of medical education and supervision of trainees in New York. The resultant committee, headed by Dr Bertrand Bell, recommended several changes. The Bell Commission proposed limitations on duty hours for trainees such that residents should not exceed an average of 80 hours per week averaged over a 4-week period with no single shift exceeding 24 hours.[20–22] These changes were formally adopted by New York in 1989. In 2003, similar duty hour policies were adopted nationwide by the Accreditation Council for Graduate Medical Education (ACGME).[20] In 2008, the Institute of Medicine published a report recommending additional restrictions on resident duty hours in an effort to further enhance safety and supervision. The ACGME subsequently convened a task force to analyze these recommendations and identified additional benefit of duty hour restriction. Additional revisions were adopted by the ACGME in 2011, which placed additional limitations on work hours for interns and mandated supervision for patient handoffs.[20,23]

The consequences of the reformation in duty hour policies have been mixed. Multiple studies have attempted to evaluate the effects of duty hour restrictions on patient safety and resident wellness with variable results. One meta-analysis suggested that duty hour restrictions had a positive effect on resident wellness based on subjective quality-of-life scores.[23] However, other survey data suggested that although the majority (61.8%) of interns reported improvement in quality of life, more senior residents reported a decrease in quality of life (49.7%) following implementation of the 2011 work hour restrictions.[24] Specifically in regard to surgical trainees, there have been mixed results of duty hours restrictions on perceived wellness with approximately half of studies reporting improvement in perceived wellness, whereas the remainder identified no change in perceived wellness.[25] In addition, this review suggests that the work hour limitations placed on interns were associated with a decreased level of professional satisfaction and preparedness for more senior roles, which may have a negative impact on burnout.

In response to the poor quality of data and mixed outcomes regarding the 2011 ACGME duty hour changes, the Flexibility in Duty Hour Requirements for Surgical Trainees (FIRST) trial was conducted. This noninferiority trial comparing the standard 2011 ACGME duty hour policies with flexible duty hour policies in surgical training programs aimed to assess patient safety along with resident satisfaction outcomes. The flexible hour policy maintained the maximum work hours of 80 hours per week averaged over 4 weeks but introduced flexibility in shift length and eliminated minimum requirements for time off between shifts. These changes attempted to address concerns regarding excessive patient handoffs and missed educational opportunities due to shift length limitations. The FIRST trial found no difference in patient outcomes between standard and flexible hour groups. Residents in the flexible work hour group reported improved satisfaction with continuity of care and surgical training; however, residents in the flexible work hour group reported a negative impact on time outside of work such as ability to spend time with family or in pursuit of extracurricular activities. Overall, there was no difference in satisfaction with work hour policies between groups.[26]

## BEYOND DUTY HOURS: TOWARD AN EMPHASIS ON PHYSICIAN WELL-BEING

The mixed results of the impact of duty hours on resident wellness suggest that resident wellness is affected by much more than time spent at work. Furthermore, in the years following surgical training, hours worked has not been associated with burnout or wellness.[27] Many factors, both on the individual and system level, have been proposed as possible determinants of wellness and burnout in training. These factors include feelings of isolation, delayed gratification associated with the length of surgical training, limited control over the practice environment, an inefficient or hostile work environment, the requirements of electronic medical records, and pressures related to patient outcomes.[27–29]

As physician burnout has been identified as contributor to worse patient outcomes, there has been increasing motivation to identify mitigating factors to burnout and the promotion of wellness. In a 2018 survey of General Surgery residents, several factors were associated with increased reports of burnout based on the MBI.[13] First, burnout was more prevalent early in training, with postgraduate year 1 (PGY-1) trainees being more likely to have symptoms of burnout than PGY-4 and PGY-5 residents. Furthermore, mistreatment, described as a composite measure of discrimination, harassment, and abuse, was associated with burnout with higher levels or burnout reported with an increasing frequency of mistreatment. Finally, there was a stepwise increase in burnout reported with increasing number of duty hour violations. These findings have led to the development of the Surgical Education Culture Optimization through targeted interventions based on National comparative Data (SECOND) trial, which is currently underway. This trial aims to further define the state current state of wellness among General Surgery residents and identify tools to improve the learning environment and resident well-being.

## WELLNESS: THE NEXT STEPS

The benefits of "being well" are obvious for not only the individual surgeon but for society in general. However, as previously described, the precise definition of wellness remains elusive, as this is an individualized concept, and therefore, achieving a pathway to wellness is likewise difficult to script. Certainly, limiting work hours and setting work-life balance are important considerations that allow for pursuit of "wellness" activities outside of the hospital, but there has to be more beyond time outside of the hospital.

For surgical educators, prioritizing wellness during training has to be an important first step in turning the unsustainable tide of surgeon burn out. Only by instilling this important aspect of self-care and self-preservation will surgeons of the future be able to meet the needs of future patients. Specific examples that are variably practiced in residency training programs are designated wellness days for "resident-free" activities that focus on team-building, teamwork, and a scheduled break from patient care responsibilities. Beyond such episodic events, encouraging healthy eating, promoting healthy sleeping, and regular exercise are systematic changes that must be emphasized by, and for, surgeons. Regular physical exercise has innumerable benefits and can be incorporated through either corporate exercise or easy access to exercise facilities within the hospital. These changes are always easier to state than to reliably incorporate into the frenetic pace of a surgeon's daily schedule; however, incremental changes that emphasize well-being have to start taking root. From a mental health perspective, increased emphasis on stress management, enhancing resiliency, and acknowledging health care specific issues, such as second victim syndrome, are all positive steps forward.[30] A commitment to further educating physicians about mental health, destigmatizing the negative connotations of "mental health," offering peer and professional support services after adverse events, and recognizing the importance of mental health in long-term wellness are possible paths forward.

Likewise, it is imperative that the principles of wellness are valued for practicing surgeons in various practice settings. The individual surgeon must introspectively identify aspects that contribute to wellness and ensure that these values are prioritized and protected. For surgeons who are in leadership roles, caring for the surgeons in their scope of responsibility should expand beyond traditional metrics and include the incorporation of well-being, which will assuredly lead to more engaged and satisfied surgeons. Moreover, although a subtle difference, we must not confuse "avoiding burnout" with "being well." The former is a passive act that is thrust on the surgeon with numerous negative implications, whereas the latter is an active state of enhancing overall happiness. To that end, surgeons must actively and habitually practice wellness-instilling pathways to continue to enjoy the satisfaction of a surgical career.

## WHAT IS RESILIENCE AND WHY DO WE CARE?

In a general sense, resilience is the tendency to adapt and succeed despite adverse conditions while maintaining the individual's well-being. With so much attention turned toward physician burn out and job satisfaction in today's health care era, the concept of resilience has made its way to the forefront of the discussion. When did resilience first become a topic of academic inquiry? Of course, throughout history, people have been captured by stories of heroic figures surmounting impossible conditions. But rigorous operationalization and scientific study of resilience was first materialized in the 1960s in child psychology and the concept has since found much application in the study of psychiatric illnesses such as posttraumatic stress disorder (PTSD) and major depressive disorder.[31]

Significant progress has subsequently been made in understanding the factors that influence the resilience of an individual. We have evolved past imagining resilience as merely the absence of maladaptive changes in the face of stress to understanding resilience as active processes along multiple domains that function to adapt the individual to challenging circumstances. Although the exact operationalization of the concept of resilience varies greatly from study to study, the overall body of literature strongly supports the notion that resilience is crucial for individuals frequently exposed to significant stressors to continue flourishing in their environments and prevent development of psychiatric illness such as depression and PTSD.[32–35] Within the field of medicine specifically, resilience has been a core research question in the investigation of provider burnout, an ever-increasing phenomenon that strips away talented minds from the profession.[36] The surgical profession is uniquely challenging, and although this provides a substrate for surgeons to thrive, it can also threaten to overwhelm them if they are not adequately equipped to confront the stressors of the job.

Resilience is best understood as a complex biopsychosocial concept, with determinants in all 3 domains that likely interact with one another on a regular basis.

## PERSONAL PSYCHOLOGICAL FACTORS

Initial conceptions of resilience were relatively limited to the psychological domain. Resilience was seen as a fixed personality trait, and as other personality traits, psychological research has mostly conducted its inquiry by means of factor analysis and questionnaires that ask subjects to report how much they identify with statements such as "I work to attain my goals," "I take a long time to get over set-backs," and "I can deal with new and unusual situations."[37] Trait theory traditionally views traits as mostly stable over time, but modern psychological research has begun to view psychological resilience as a more dynamic and adaptive phenomenon that can be nurtured or neglected.[38] Most likely, other psychological traits, as well as biological and social factors, work to constantly affect an individual's trait resilience. Whatever the case, research has clearly shown that high levels of trait resilience are protective against negative mental health outcomes.[39] Trait resilience has been correlated with other well-established psychological traits such as extraversion, openness, agreeableness, and conscientiousness and negatively correlated with neuroticism, that is, the tendency toward anxiety and negative emotions.[40]

A key psychological factor that has come to the forefront of resilience is the concept of moral injury. First introduced by psychiatrist Jonathan Shay, moral injury was originally used in the context of psychologically traumatized Vietnam War veterans. Shay observed that veterans who had experienced events that violated their deeply held moral convictions were more likely to develop PTSD.[41] These become deep wounds in the soul that "undoes" a person's character. For many health care providers, entering the field of medicine is the actualization of a deeply held conviction that improving the lives of other human beings is a personal calling and moral obligation. With this in mind, many researchers are now investigating whether the realities of the modern health care system produce significant moral injury by undermining physicians' sense of efficacy in affecting the positive change they set off to produce in their careers. A Rand Corporation survey on physician burnout found that the primary stressor affecting responding physicians was the inability to provide accessible, high-quality, and affordable health care.[42] Understandably, the motivation to continue working in an inherently stressful environment deteriorates when, instead of actively caring for patients, providers are spending hours navigating tedious electronic systems, insurance requirements, and medicolegal threats. When a patient suffers a negative outcome from something we feel we should have been able to control but could not, this can be a profound source of moral injury.

Another crucial psychological factor that has received much attention is empathy and compassion fatigue. Empathy and compassion are related concepts, both generally referring to the ability to feel the suffering that another being is experiencing and the desire to alleviate that suffering.[43] Providers have finite reserves of emotional energy to provide to patients. When that limit has been reached, compassion fatigue sets in and works to emotionally distance provider from patient. Research has shown that compassion fatigue and trait resilience are qualities that both affect each other.[44]

## SOCIAL FACTORS

As alluded to previously, initial inquiry into resilience focused on child development, and our understanding of social determinants of resilience owes much to that body of work. Secure maternal attachments, family stability, and strong peer support are classically associated with development of strong resilience.[45] But do modifiable social factors still play a role in adult surgeons? The answer is a resounding yes. Nontoxic work environments that promote positive self-esteem, provide exciting opportunities, and responsibly mitigate risk of negative consequences have all been linked to improved resilience against adverse conditions. Anecdotal reports have described the positive effect of strong role models and mentors in reinforcing resilience of trainees.[46] Sense of control over the work schedule, fair evaluation, balance between reward and effort, an ability to cultivate personal hobbies outside of work, and a feeling of belonging to the community of fellow colleagues both inside and outside of work are all factors that improve resilience.[47] Conversely, poor team communication, clinical data overload, time pressures, lack of appropriate clinical resources, and lack of leisure time (ie, work-life balance) are associated with impaired resilience and increased burnout.[48]

## INSTILLING RESILIENCE

Although resilience is widely recognized as a necessary quality for surgeons, mechanisms for instilling resilience have not been widely studied. Most of the discussion on this topic relies on extrapolation from pediatric observational studies, which themselves have not identified a reproducible approach for instilling resilience in children. Nevertheless, what seems clear is that resilience develops through overcoming adversity,[49] with the ability to do so depending on a delicate balance between the individual and the environment.

It therefore stands to reason that many surgeons feel formal resilience training is superfluous, as the rigorous gauntlet for acceptance into, and graduation from, surgical residency is itself an adequate process. Those who overcome adversity either have or develop resilience matriculate, whereas those who do not or cannot remove themselves from training. Although this may be true in some instances, the very method we rely on for developing resilience is not standardized and in many cases minimally supervised. This means we have passively allowed many fantastic residents to burn out in programs where the environment does not optimize the individual's ability to develop resiliency. Furthermore, it clearly has failed, as an exceedingly high burnout rate exists among both residents and fully trained surgeons.[28]

In spite of the obvious difficulties and the complexity of the issue, there is an opportunity to address the issue of resilience among surgeons. We have already made note of some of the specific challenges facing surgeons, but how do we intervene to improve resiliency? In one survey study of faculty within a Department of Medicine, physicians who spent at least 20% of their time in the aspect of work that was most meaningful to them had a rate of burnout nearly half that of those who spent less than 20%.[50] Of course, the implication is that the surgeons understand what aspect of surgical care brings joy and then make it a point that this joyful activity is protected and continued on a regular basis. Other purposeful activities that have been suggested to enhance resilience includes cultivating relationships with peers; developing hobbies outside of work; developing a sense of community of peers, volunteer work, or community service; and developing mindfulness.

Resilience can be affected on personal and organizational levels. On a personal level, in addition to aforementioned activities, ensuring personal health to include regular health care appointments with a qualified (not another surgeon) physician, exercising regularly, and healthy eating all contribute to overall well-being and thus, resilience. On an organizational level, the ideal actions to enhance resilience remain elusive. One meta-analysis suggested that structural changes, fostering communication between members of the health care team, and cultivating a sense of teamwork are the mainstays of developing organizational resilience and furthermore, more effective than physician-directed interventions[51];this suggests that such changes from an organizational level are more effective, yet more complex in ensuring the overall mental health of the providers.

## SUMMARY

Wellness and resilience are key components of a successful and fulfilling surgical career. Although we cannot completely reset surgeon and hospital culture, we can promote wellness and resilience in tangible ways. Although this will require a cultural shift among surgeons that is long over-due, this shift will ultimately turn the tide of surgeon burn out. Emphasizing the importance of wellness and enabling self-efficacy, confidence, and perseverance must begin immediately at all levels but should also be emphasized to the future surgeon work force during residency training. Across the entire spectrum of surgical care delivery, we must choose to pass on our lessons learned; supply actionable feedback; and promote a culture of teamwork, mutual respect, and empathy. With a little extra effort, we can influence our culture in a way that sustains each other and our profession through any adversity.

## DISCLOSURE

The views expressed herein are those of the author and do not reflect the official policy or position of Madigan Army Medical Center, the US Army Medical Department, the Department of Defense, or the US Government.

## REFERENCES

1. Lebares CC, Guvva EV, Ascher NL, et al. Burnout and stress among us surgery residents: psychological distress and resilience. J Am Coll Surg 2018;226(1): 80–90.
2. Shanafelt TD, West CP, Sinsky C, et al. Changes in burnout and satisfaction with work-life integration in physicians and the general US working population between 2011 and 2017. Mayo Clin Proc 2019;94(9):1681–94.
3. Dyrbye LN, West CP, Satele D, et al. Burnout among U.S. medical students, residents, and early career physicians relative to the general U.S. population. Acad Med 2014;89(3):443–51.
4. History of Wellness. Global wellness institute. Available at: https://globalwellnessinstitute.org/industry-research/history-of-wellness/. Accessed October 15, 2020.
5. Miller G, Foster LT. Critical synthesis of wellness literature. Heal Promot. 2010;(February):1-32. Available at: https://dspace.library.uvic.ca:8443/handle/1828/2894. Accessed October 12, 2020.
6. Dunn HL. High-level wellness for man and society. Am J Public Health 1959; 49(6):786–92.
7. Dunn HL. High level wellness, Vol 53. Arlington, Virginia: RW Beatty, LTD; 1961.
8. Shanafelt TD, Balch CM, Bechamps GJ, et al. Burnout and career satisfaction among American surgeons. Ann Surg 2009;250(3):463–70.
9. Elmore LC, Jeffe DB, Jin L, et al. National survey of burnout among US general surgery residents. J Am Coll Surg 2016;223(3):440–51.
10. Shanafelt TD, Hasan O, Dyrbye LN, et al. Changes in burnout and satisfaction with work-life balance in physicians and the general US working population between 2011 and 2014. Mayo Clin Proc 2015;90(12):1600–13.
11. Maslach C, Jackson SE. The measurement of experienced burnout. J Occup Behav 1981;2:99–113.
12. Dyrbye LN, Burke SE, Hardeman RR, et al. Association of clinical specialty with symptoms of burnout and career choice regret among US resident physicians. JAMA 2018;320(11):1114–30.
13. Hu YY, Ellis RJ, Hewitt DB, et al. Discrimination, abuse, harassment, and burnout in surgical residency training. N Engl J Med 2019;381(18):1741–52.
14. Shanafelt TD, Balch CM, Dyrbye L, et al. Special report: suicidal ideation among American surgeons. Arch Surg 2011;146(1):54–62.
15. Oreskovich MR, Shanafelt T, Dyrbye LN, et al. The prevalence of substance use disorders in American physicians. Am J Addict 2015;24(1):30–8.
16. Wallace JE, Lemaire JB, Ghali WA. Physician wellness: a missing quality indicator. Lancet 2009. https://doi.org/10.1016/S0140-6736(09)61424-0.
17. Shanafelt TD, Noseworthy JH. Executive leadership and physician well-being: nine organizational strategies to promote engagement and reduce burnout. Mayo Clin Proc 2017;92(1):129–46.
18. Oaklander M. Doctors on life support. TIME Mag. 2015. Available at: https://time.com/4012840/doctors-on-life-support/. Accessed October 12, 2020.

19. Lerner BH. A life-changing case for doctors in training. The New York Times. 2009. Available at: https://www.nytimes.com/2009/03/03/health/03zion.html. Accessed October 12, 2020.
20. Fabricant PD, Dy CJ, Dare DM, et al. A narrative review of surgical resident duty hour limits: where do we go from here? J Grad Med Educ 2013;5(1):19–24.
21. Frishman WH, Alpert JS. Reform in house staff working hours and clinical supervision: a 30-year reflection following the release of the bell commission report. Am J Med 2018;131(12):1399–400.
22. Bell BM. Supervision, not regulation of hours, is the key to improving the quality of patient care. JAMA 1993;269(3):403–4.
23. Lin H, Lin E, Auditore S, et al. A narrative review of high-quality literature on the effects of resident duty hours reforms. Acad Med 2016;91(1):140–50.
24. Drolet BC, Derrick CA, Fischer SA. Residents' response to duty-hour regulations-a follow-up national survey. N Engl J Med 2012;366(24):e35.
25. Ahmed N, Devitt KS, Keshet I, et al. A systematic review of the effects of resident duty hour restrictions in surgery: Impact on resident wellness, training, and patient outcomes. Ann Surg 2014;259(6):1041–53.
26. Bilimoria KY, Chung JW, Hedges LV, et al. National cluster-randomized trial of duty-hour flexibility in surgical training. N Engl J Med 2016;374:713–27.
27. Balch CM, Freischlag JA, Shanafelt TD. Stress and burnout among surgeons. Arch Surg 2009;144(4):371.
28. Patti MG, Schlottmann F, Sarr MG. The problem of burnout among surgeons. JAMA Surg 2018;153(5):403–4.
29. Pulcrano M, Evans SRT, Sosin M. Quality of life and burnout rates across surgical specialties: a systematic review. JAMA Surg 2016;151(10):970–8.
30. Wu A. Medical error: the second victim. The doctor who makes the mistake needs help too. BMJ 2000;320(7237):726–7.
31. Masten AS. Resilience in developing systems: progress and promise as the fourth wave rises. Dev Psychopathol 2007;19:921–30.
32. Rakesh G, Morey RA, Zannas AS, et al. Resilience as a translational endpoint in the treatment of PTSD. Mol Psychiatry 2019;24:1268–83.
33. Horn SR, Charney DS, Feder A. Understanding resilience: new approaches for preventing and treating PTSD. Exp Neurol 2016;284(Pt B):119–32.
34. Edward K. Resilience: a protector from depression. Am Psy Nurse Assoc 2005; 11(4):241–3.
35. Laird KT, Krause B, Funes C, et al. Psychobiological factors of resilience and depression in late life. Translational Psychiatry 2019;9(1):1–18.
36. West CP, Dyrbye LN, Sinsky C, et al. Resilience and burnout among physicians and the general us working population. JAMA Netw Open 2020;3(7):e209385.
37. Maltby J, Day L, Hall S. Refining trait resilience: identifying engineering, ecological, and adaptive facets from extant measures of resilience. PLoS One 2015; 10(7):e0131826.
38. Leys C, Arnal C, Wollast R, et al. Perspectives on resilience: personality trait or skill? Eur J Trauma Dissoc 2020;4(2):100074.
39. Hu T, Zhang D, Wang J. A meta-analysis of the trait resilience and mental health. Personal Individual Differences 2015;76:18–27.
40. Oshio A, Taku K, Hirano M, et al. Resilience and big five personality traits: a meta-analysis. Personal Individual Differences 2018;127:54–60.
41. Shay J. Achilles in Vietnam: combat trauma and the undoing of character. Oxford, New York: Maxwell Macmillan International, Atheneum; 1994.

42. Rozario D. Burnout, resilience and moral injury: how the wicked problems of health care defy solutions, yet require innovative strategies in the modern era. Can J Surg 2019;62(4):E6–8.

43. Goetz JL, Keltner D, Simon-Thomas E. Compassion: an evolutionary analysis and empirical review. Psychol Bull 2010;136(3):351–74.

44. Figley CR, Figley KR. In: Seppälä EM, Simon-Thomas E, Brown SL, et al, editors. Compassion fatigue resilience, vol. 1. Oxford University Press; 2017.

45. Herrman H, Stewart DE, Diaz-Granados N, et al. What is resilience? Can J Psychiatry 2011;56(5):258–65.

46. Abaza MM, Nelson KG. Leading by example: role modeling resilience helps our learners and ourselves. Acad Med 2018;93(2):157–8.

47. Jennings ML, Slavin SJ. Resident wellness matters: optimizing resident education and wellness through the learning environment. Acad Med 2015;90(9):1246–50.

48. Matheson C, Robertson HD, Elliott AM, et al. Resilience of primary healthcare professionals working in challenging environments: a focus group study. Br J Gen Pract 2016;66(648):e507–15.

49. Howe A, Smajdor A, Stockl A. Towards an understanding of resilience and its relevance to medical training. Med Educ 2012;46:349–56.

50. Shanafelt TD, West CP, Sloan JA, et al. Career fit and burnout among academic faculty. Arch Intern Med 2009;169(10):990–5.

51. Panagioti M, Panagopoulou E, Bower P, et al. Controlled interventions to reduce burnout in physicians. JAMA Intern Med 2017;177(2):195–205.

# Medical Student Selection

Ian Kratzke, MD[a], Muneera R. Kapadia, MD, MME[b],
Fumiko Egawa, MD[c], Jennifer S. Beaty, MD[d],*

## KEYWORDS

- Medical students • Medical schools • Admissions • Selection • MCAT • GPA
- Personal statement • Interviews

## KEY POINTS

- Medical school admissions rely heavily on The Medical College Admissions Test and grade point averages to evaluate applicants.
- Personal statements and letters of recommendation evaluations are not standardized and their usefulness is unclear.
- Interviews for medical school are moving to multiple mini interview models with rapid adoption of virtual interviews in the era of coronavirus disease 2019.
- Medical schools show little progress with increasing diversity of students.

## INTRODUCTION

Selecting medical students is an incredibly important responsibility because it shapes the future of the medical profession. Medical students represent a huge investment as it takes years to train individuals from the beginning of medical school to the completion of graduate medical education. They are an important potential societal resource, because they will care for our future ailing patients. Our physician workforce must be prepared to serve an increasingly diverse community. Therefore, racial, ethnic, and gender diversity among our future physicians is paramount for relating to patients. We must strive to select students with not only diverse backgrounds and experiences, but also with diverse interests and strengths to fill all the necessary niches within the broad field of medicine. In addition to future clinicians, some will be educators, teaching the students and residents of the future; some will be researchers, pushing the science of medicine forward; and some will be leaders, guiding organizations and the business of medicine. Being granted admission to medical school is a privilege and selecting medical students should be approached with care and thoughtfulness.

[a] The University of North Carolina at Chapel Hill, Department of Surgery, 4001 Burnett-Womack Building, CB #7050, 101 Manning Drive, Chapel Hill, NC 27599-7050, USA; [b] The University of North Carolina at Chapel Hill, Department of Surgery, 4038 Burnett-Womack Building, 101 Manning Drive, Chapel Hill, NC 27599-7081, USA; [c] Creighton University, Department of Surgery, Education Building, Ste. 501, 7710 Mercy Road, Omaha, NE 68124-2386, USA; [d] Des Moines University College of Osteopathic Medicine, 3200 Grand Avenue, #148, Des Moines, IA 50312, USA
* Corresponding author.
E-mail address: Jennifer.Beaty@dmu.edu

Surg Clin N Am 101 (2021) 635–652
https://doi.org/10.1016/j.suc.2021.05.010
0039-6109/21/© 2021 Elsevier Inc. All rights reserved.
surgical.theclinics.com

## GRADUATION AND ATTRITION OF MEDICAL STUDENTS

Determining medical student selection is somewhat variable depending on the priorities of individual institutions. However, metrics available in the United States indicate that the students admitted to medical school are generally successful. The American Association of Medical Colleges (AAMC) reports 4-year graduation rates have been stable, between 82% to 84%, and 96% of students finish by 6 years after matriculation.[1] The US Medical License Examination (USMLE) pass rates are similarly high for first-time examinees with an MD degree; in 2018 and 2019, the individual board examination pass rates were as follows: 96% to 97% for USMLE 1, 97% to 98% for USMLE 2 Clinical Knowledge, 95% for USMLE 2 Clinical Skills, and 98% for USMLE 3.[2] Of the students entering the national residency match program in 2020, 91% matched into their preferred residency specialty. Surgical applicants had overall lower match rates, ranging between 72% and 83%, depending on the surgical subspecialty.[3]

In 1965, the AAMC reported medical school attrition was 9%.[4] More recently, much lower attrition rates have has been reported, approximately 3% per year over the last 20 years, with most students citing nonacademic reasons for leaving medical school.[1] However, a systematic review published in 2011 found struggling academically may be strongly associated with medical student dropout.[5] In 2007, a report released by the AAMC demonstrated attrition rates differed by race/ethnicity, with Black, African American, Native American, Hispanic, and Latino students having higher attrition rates than White and Asian students.[6] Additionally, medical students from lower socioeconomic status backgrounds were also more likely to leave medical school in the first 2 years.[7] Although the great majority of medical students graduate, attrition is costly to the individual students, medical schools, and society at large; therefore, there is a collective interest to select students who will be successful.

### *Medical School Applications*

The American Medical College Application Service serves as a centralized application processing service and most US medical schools use the American Medical College Application Service application as their primary application.[8] Some medical schools have additional secondary applications that contain specific questions pertinent to the individual institutions. Finally, most schools have an interview component to the application process. The individual components to the application (**Table 1**) and their effects on medical student selection and performance are discussed elsewhere in this article.

| Table 1 Medical school application process | | |
| --- | --- | --- |
| **AMCAS Application** | **Secondary Application** | **Interview** |
| Sociodemographics | School-specific essays | Institution specific |
| Education | | |
| MCAT | | |
| Extracurricular experiences | | |
| Personal statement | | |
| LORs | | |

*Abbreviations:* ASMCAS, American Medical College Application Service; MCAT, Medical College Admission Test.

## Sociodemographics

The demographics of applicants to medical school have experienced significant changes over the past 40 years, with an increase from approximately 36,000 total applicants per year, to now approximately 53,000 applicants per year.[9] In the past 5 years, however, the number of applicants has remained relatively stable, and the matriculation rate has increased steadily.[10]

### Age and gender

The age of applicants has remained stable over the past few years, with an average age of 24 years old, and is similar for both men and women applicants.[11] The gender of applicants historically has been majority male; however, in the early 2000s there was a decrease in male applicants as compared with female applicants.[12,13] This trend led to a fairly equal number of male and female applicants, until the 2017–2018 application cycle, which saw for the first time fewer male applicants as compared with female applicants, and this trend has continued.[12]

### Minority status

Over the last 4 application cycles, the numbers of under-represented minorities (URM) has increased slightly, with the greatest increase in Asian and Hispanic applicants, and a steady number of Black or African American applicants.[14] White applicants remain the largest proportion of total applicants to medical school; however, the numbers of White applicants has decreased in the last year.[14]

There has been a national effort to increase the representation of minorities within medical schools, with a range of strategies for increasing minority representation.[15] The factors that have been shown to increase the likelihood of minorities applying to medical school include elementary school success, parental influence, and financial support.[13] Specifically, the success of African American men applying to medical school may be related to prior exposure to medicine and a strong social support system.[16]

The performance of URM applicants before medical school has been shown to be different as compared with White applicants, with URM students having lower admissions scores based on their academic performance.[17] Although URM students may have lower grades in the gateway courses for application to medical school, they have a higher completion rate of these undergraduate courses when compared with White students.[18] Finally, adjusting the admission's criteria from grade based to attribute based to increase the diversity of selected students has not been shown to improve admission rates for URM.[19] However, by creating a more holistic application process that is less focused on grades does increase the diversity of students interviewed for medical school.

### Disparities

There are also certain characteristics of applicants that affect application rates and acceptance rates to medical school outside of undergraduate performance. Notably, there is a selection bias for applicants with parents who are doctors, even though they may have lower examination scores.[20] Additionally, the geographic setting of applicants seems to play a role in the likelihood of applying to medical school. Although applicants from both rural and urban areas demonstrate similar undergraduate scores and have similar admission rates, there are fewer rural students applying to medical school as compared with applicants from urban areas.[21,22]

## Education

### Grade point average

The undergraduate grade point average (GPA) is historically weighted heavily as a fundamental criterion for the admission decision to medical school. There has been a slight increase in the average GPA of medical school applicants over the past 4 application cycles, from 3.56 to 3.60.[23] As such, when a medical school interviewer knows the applicant's GPA, it has been shown to lead to higher interview scores, even though the GPA is not a direct component of those scores.[24] More recently, however, the importance of GPA in the admissions process has been highly debated, with arguments made that medical schools place too much emphasis on this factor. However, the majority of data suggest that the GPA does, to a varying degree, correlate with medical school performance.[25–28] The greatest correlation between undergraduate GPA and medical school performance is seen in the early years of medical school, where performance is largely measured by test taking rather than clinical skill.[29] It is less clear, however, if student performance in the preclinical years of medical school translates to their performance during the clinical years of medical school.[30] Finally, there are data suggesting a correlation between undergraduate GPA and USMLE scores, especially USMLE Step 1.[31]

### Major

Most medical schools require the completion of certain undergraduate classes; however, these requirements vary based on the school.[32] Premedical requisite classes are typically related to the sciences and, therefore, most applicants are those with biological science majors, making up 58% of applicants during the 2020–2021 cycle.[33] Within this same application cycle, 28% of applicants were nonscience majors, indicating that these students remain a significant percentage of the applicant pool.[33] Nonscience major applicants have been shown to experience less of a sense of preparedness in applying to medical school and lower scores in early training.[34]

### Undergraduate institutions

The type of undergraduate program that applicants apply from is also an area of interest to medical schools. Most notably, attending a private undergraduate college may improve the likelihood of admission to medical school, independent of their academic performance.[35] Additionally, for African American applicants, attending an historically Black university or college improves the likelihood of admission to medical school.[36] There is also evidence that medical students who attended liberal arts colleges tend to have lower medical school grades as compared with university graduates; however, liberal arts graduates are more likely to be accepted in to honorary organizations such as the Alpha Omega Alpha society.[37] Finally, although there has not been shown to be differences in performance for applicants from community-focused colleges, these students have demonstrated higher levels of agreeableness and conscientiousness based on study data.[38]

### Graduate degrees

The most common graduate degree of students applying to medical school are premedical preparatory degrees, termed postbaccalaureate premedical programs or special masters programs. These courses are designed to enhance applicants' preparedness for medical school and increase their chances of admission. Approximately 15% of matriculants to medical school previously acquired such a degree.[39] Although these degrees may lead to additional time and expenses for the applicant, they have been shown to be successful in increasing the diversity of the matriculant class, because a disproportionate number of postbaccalaureate premedical program graduates include URMs.[40] Importantly, these same applicants have been shown to be more likely to practice in underserved areas as physicians.[39]

*Medical College Admissions Test Scores*

*Correlation with board scores*

In addition to the applicants' GPA, The Medical College Admissions Test (MCAT) scores remain a fundamental aspect of admission criteria for medical school. Average total MCAT scores over the last 4 application cycles has increased from 504.7 to 506.4.[23] There has been extensive research into the correlation of MCAT scores and subsequent medical student success, with general agreement that there is at least some correlation between MCAT scores and USMLE scores.[31,41–43] This finding is particularly true for USMLE Step 1 scores.[44] As for medical school performance, MCAT scores have not been shown to correlate with this measure.[25,27] However, MCAT scores do correlate with success in graduating from medical school.[45]

There are a few exceptions to the correlation between MCAT scores and USMLE scores. Specifically, the verbal reasoning scores are less predictive of board scores when English is not the primary language of the student.[46] Additionally, students who require accommodations for completing the MCAT owing to disabilities may have lower board scores than would be expected when compared with their MCAT scores.[47] Finally, and in contrast with the trends seen with GPA scores, when a medical school interviewer is aware of the applicant's MCAT score, there does not seem to be an influence on their interview score.[24]

*Disparities between age, sex, race, and socioeconomic status*

The relationship between MCAT scores and applicant demographics remains a topic of interest for medical schools. In terms of gender, male applicants on average have higher MCAT scores without differences in GPA or medical school performance as compared with female applicants.[48] Additionally, when medical schools accept more midrange MCAT scores, this factor has been shown to lead to an increase in the diversity of the matriculating class.[49] Finally, there is evidence that applicants from underdeveloped or rural areas may have lower MCAT scores,[50] but that participation in MCAT preparatory courses may improve rural students' scores and subsequently encourage practice in underserved communities.[51]

*Reapplicants*

*Changes to the application*

After significant investment in applying to medical school, some applicants, unfortunately, do not receive an admission. This factor leads to a pool of applicants who are considered reapplicants and who must now compete with first-time applicants. Overall, most reapplicants demonstrate improvements in test scores and admission scores, leading to higher admission rates than first-time applicants.[52]

*Matriculation success rate*

Students who choose to reapply to medical school are typically those with higher initial undergraduate scores and are less likely to be from a rural area.[52] If, however, applicants had an alternative graduate degree program plan, they were less likely to reapply to medical school.[53] Additionally, if they had high education debt, they were also less likely to reapply, suggesting an inability to afford the process.[53]

*Extracurricular Experience*

Extracurricular experience is a key aspect of medical school admission scores, yet its weight in the admission decision varies by school. Female applicants typically report greater participation in extracurricular activities.[54] Those with more extracurricular activity experience before medical school are more likely to demonstrate persistent extracurricular activities during medical school, and additionally have higher medical school performance.[55] In contrast, liberal arts students tend to participate in fewer extracurricular activities during medical school but are more likely to be in honorary organizations such as the American Osteopathic Association.[37]

### Patient exposure

Although most medical school applicants have no prior experience in health care, a proportion of applicants come from another branch in the health care industry. Importantly, these applicants with prior medical training have higher percentages of matriculation.[20] If there is no direct experience in health care, shadowing practicing physicians is one way applicants may demonstrate exposure to the health care field.

### Research

Research is another area of the medical school admission score whose weight varies by school, and applicants who participate in premedical research programs have higher medical school acceptance rates, even with lower GPAs.[56]

### Community service

Community service is another aspect of extracurricular activities considered by admission scores. For applicants who are women, who volunteered at multiple types of organizations, and who participated in these service opportunities for more than 2 years, they are shown to be more likely to pursue community service opportunities while in medical school.[57]

## PERSONAL STATEMENT

The personal statement requires medical school applicants to describe themselves in a brief and unique essay. Premedical programs place an emphasis on beginning writing the statement early, continually rewriting it, and reflecting deeply on what to write about.[58] This aspect of the application causes a level of discomfort and stress for applicants, because it requires skills not necessarily seen elsewhere in the application, which has led to a concerning number of applicants plagiarizing.[59] In contrast with the focus placed on the personal statement before applying, admission committees have not been shown to weigh this aspect of the application heavily; in fact, it is typically viewed as one of the least important aspects of the application by those making the application decision.[60,61] One reason for this finding may be that the evidence for the predictive validity of personal statements on the success of medical students is weak and varied.[62] Personal statements have been seen as a tool to measure the interpersonal skills of applicants; however, they have not been shown to fulfill this goal.[63] Although medical schools continue to require personal statements from their applicants, the criteria used for evaluating them are not standardized and their usefulness remains unclear.[62]

## SCHOOL-SPECIFIC ESSAYS

There is a paucity of research on whether secondary application essays are valid indicators of medical students' future performance. Dong and colleagues[64] designed a study that demonstrated that none of the medical school performance indicators were significantly correlated with the essay scores. This finding calls into question the usefulness of matriculation essays, a resource-intensive admission requirement. Furthermore, the fee structure for secondary applications can also add up quickly. Students are required to pay up to US$150 for secondary applications per school.[65] In 2019, 36.7% of those entering medical school spent more than US $2000 on secondary applications.[66] Because the validity is marginal at best and significant costs exist, secondary applications should not be sent out until adequate screening of the applicants is completed.

## SOCIAL MEDIA

Little is known about the use of social media and its role in medical school admissions. The AAMC has a statement on their webpage "how social media can affect your application."[67] Students are advised to assume the admissions committees do look up applicants online.

## LETTERS OF RECOMMENDATION

Letters of recommendation (LORs) are a standard component of a medical school application. According to American Medical College Application Service guidelines, students may upload multiple letters and select which letters to send to which schools.[8] Letters may be written by undergraduate faculty, employers, and supervisors, among others. These LORs, as part of a holistic review, are intended to strengthen an application by demonstrating how an applicant's personal characteristics are indicative of future success in medical school and beyond.[68] LORs may indicate whether a candidate has the grit or hardiness that, in conjunction with a disadvantaged background, has been considered an indirect indicator of future success.[69] However, there is room for interpretation of LORs owing in part to variability in content, structure, and letter writers themselves. There is also an associated cost in time spent by the admissions committee reviewing LORs.[62]

The literature suggests that LORs do not predict performance in medical school consistently.[62,70,71] In a unique attempt to try to answer the age-old LOR question, DeZee and associates[70] designed a study to assess newly graduated medical students in the top and bottom of the class and re-review their initial LORs by blind reviewers. After reviewing 437 LORs for 76 unique characteristics, only a few characteristics were actually helpful. Being rated as "the best" among peers and having an employer or supervisor as the LOR author were both associated with being in the top of the class, whereas a nonpositive comment was associated with being in the bottom of the class. The authors concluded LORs have limited value to admission committees, because very few LOR characteristics predict how students perform during medical school.[70]

Currently, there is not a standardized format for LORs as part of the medical school application. Owing to the free-form nature, it may be difficult to interpret letters and use them effectively to differentiate between 2 candidates. Albanese and colleagues[72] proposed the use of a standard letter format or the development of national guidelines for letters, either of which would help to increase the ease of evaluation by the admissions committee. They go further and propose the use of an electronic letters system to address concerns of fraudulent letters, including letters written by an applicant and signed by the letter writer or text copied from a previously written letter for a successful applicant.[72] The consensus suggests that LORs provide little added value to an application because the content of the letters do not predict student performance.[73]

## INTERVIEW PROCESS

The interview process is a standard component of medical school applications, whether to allopathic, osteopathic, or offshore medical school programs. GPA and MCAT scores are the 2 most common screening tools used by the admissions committee to evaluate to whom an interview invitation should be extended. The interview itself serves multiple purposes: for the applicant to collect data on a particular program or institution, for the applicant and program alike to present a human side during an otherwise impersonal process, and for programs to evaluate an applicant's communication skills and noncognitive abilities. Interview formats vary widely, from a traditional one-to-one interview that may range from structured questions to free-form dialogue, to a panel interview, to the highly structured objective structured clinical examination-style multiple mini interview format. The use of interviews, traditional or a multiple mini interview format, virtual or in-person, is listed as one means of achieving a holistic review of the applicant (AAMC).[74]

The validity of interviews is questionable at best. Traditional interviews have not consistently demonstrated positive predictive validity, with the exception of applicants rated extremely highly or extremely poorly.[73] Traditional interviews with structured questions are more reliable when interviewers are provided with training, standardized questions, and a rating system.[72] A recent multidisciplinary meta-analytic study to evaluate fairness and validity of interviews and holistic reviews in medical school admissions was conducted with 33 studies included.[75] The interview reliability (approximately 0.42) was low to moderate, which significantly limits its validity. This finding has been confirmed by more than 100 studies examining interview validity that collectively show interview scores to be only moderately correlated with important outcome variables.[75]

### The Multiple Mini Interview

Since the MMI was piloted and validated at McMaster University, its popularity has grown with incorporation into the admissions processes of medical schools throughout the United States and globally. The MMI scores for medical school admissions positively predicted communication skills in clinical scenarios like objective structured clinical examination performance, and GPA was the most consistent predictor of performance on multiple-choice question examinations of medical knowledge.[76] The MMI significantly predicted clinical decision-making in the objective structured clinical examination, which was not predicted by other noncognitive assessments or undergraduate GPA.[77] There was no difference in score leniency based on interviewer and applicant gender.[78] Overall, the MMI was well-accepted with a high internal reliability with an optimal number of stations and s well-structured scoring system.[79,80] The MMI use is supported as a means of decreasing bias in the selection of medical school candidates.[81] In addition, the inclusion of a writing station in the MMI allows for the evaluation of applicant communication skills that may otherwise not be tested in an interview setting. The cost and logistics MMI interviews are offset by optimizing the number of stations and interviewers.[82]

Barriers have been identified with the MMI process. They include cultural and language barriers between interviewers and applicants, and logistic feasibility.[80,83] Unfortunately, the MMI did not always increase the diversity of applicants offered interviews or admissions because the MMI alone cannot undo the diversity-limiting effects of the GPA.[84,85]

### Situational Judgment Tests

Computer-based Assessment for Sampling Personal characteristics (CASPer) is an on-line, video-based screening test. It is an situational judgment test made up of 12 sections with a video-based or word-based scenario with 3 open-ended questions. CASPer assesses collaboration, communication, empathy, equity, ethics, motivation, problem solving, professionalism, resilience, and self-awareness.[86] The inclusion of an situational judgment test such as CASPer in the admissions process has the potential to widen access to medical education for URMs.[87] The incorporation of situational judgment test as an additional nonacademic evaluation may assist medical schools with a more holistic review of applicants while observing social distancing recommendations in the time of a pandemic.[88] Further research is needed to determine the predictive validity and future role of video situational judgment test in medical school admissions.[73]

## Use of Patients

Patients have been invited to participate in a novel structured interview process. The response was very positive for the patients as well as for the applicants.[89]

## Personality Traits

The association between perfectionism and depression in the medical profession can ultimately influence physicians' performance negatively. In medical students, maladaptive perfectionism relates to distress and lower academic performance. In a review of 22 studies on personality, the big five traits (openness, conscientiousness, extroversion, agreeableness, and neuroticism) may correlate with various aspects of medical school performance.[62] Computerized personality test incorporation in the interview process has demonstrated significantly higher personality traits of honesty–humility, extraversion, agreeableness, and openness to experience, and lower traits in emotionality.[90] There is no significant correlation between personality tests and the MMI, and personality measures as a part of the selection process may not be predictive of noncognitive skills.[91] Emotional intelligence was correlated with some, but not all, measures of success during medical school matriculation and none of the measures associated with medical school admissions.[92]

## Video Conference Role

Technology is now integral to the administration of multiple admissions tools, including the Medical College Admission Test, situational judgment tests, and standardized video interviews. Consequently, today's admissions landscape is transforming into an online, globally interconnected marketplace for health professions admissions tools.[93] Asynchronous video format applications are increasing in popularity. A recent student demonstrated video conference tools can adequately evaluate leadership, innovation, social change, and creativity.[94]

Before the coronavirus disease 2019 pandemic, only 3 of 147 US allopathic programs offered video conference or telephone interviews in lieu of an in-person interview on campus. The University of New Mexico's experience with video conference interviews found no difference in the diversity of applicants admitted based on interview modality. This technology allowed for increased faculty involvement by rural and community physicians who would otherwise be unable to interview applicants owing to distance and clinical duties.[95] In light of the coronavirus disease 2019 pandemic and efforts to limit face-to-face contact, the AAMC has launched a new video interview assessment tool intended to be used in conjunction with other selection criteria and not in lieu of an in-person (or virtual) interview at any specific medical school. The Video Interview Tool for Admissions is a 1-time interview in which applicants must answer 6 questions designed to evaluate the core competencies as a part of the holistic review outlined by the AAMC.[96] Any applicant invited to interview is asked to also complete the Video Interview Tool for Admissions interview, which is then accessible to all other programs to which the applicant applied. This process is intended to support the medical schools' admission trend toward a holistic review of an applicant and the evaluation of personal characteristics that may be missed by other components of the application.

Importantly, 45% of medical school matriculants in 2019 reported spending more than $1000 on interview-related expenses alone.[66] With the transition to virtual interviewing, this change may make some institutions more accessible, although schools should remain cognizant of different means of accessing technology.[88] Further research is needed to look at the cost effectiveness of virtual interviews and their impact on the diversity of future medical school classes, because this factor significantly decreases the cost of applying to medical school for applicants and may remove a barrier for those applicants who self-select as an URM or coming from a disadvantaged background.

### The Impact of Blinding the Interviewers from the Medical College Admissions Test and Grade Point Average

Although MCAT scores accounted for some variation in interview scores for both cohorts, only access to GPA significantly influenced interviewers' scores when looking at interaction effects. Withholding academic metrics from interviewers' files may promote an assessment of nonacademic characteristics independently from academic metrics.[24]

### Applicant Preference

In a systematic literature review, applicants generally support interviews and MMIs, judging them to be relevant and fair.[80,83] Applicants felt the MMI structure eliminated cultural, gender, and age bias, and assessed noncognitive skills more effectively.[83] In the cases where a hybrid format of traditional and MMI interviews were introduced, applicants rated the MMI portions positively in voluntary postinterview surveys.[97] Applicants generally did not support panel interviews as a part of the traditional format, citing that the imbalance of numbers of faculty to applicant seems intimidating; women and persons of color are particularly critical of the use of panel formats.[72]

There is emerging evidence that situational judgment tests are also well-regarded, but aptitude tests less so. Aptitude tests and academic records were valued in decisions of whom to call to interview. Medical students prefer interview-based selection over cognitive aptitude tests.[80]

## DIFFERENCES IN APPLICATION TO TYPE OF MEDICAL SCHOOL

There is a paucity of literature comparing applicants to US allopathic programs, US osteopathic programs, and offshore medical schools. In 2008, approximately two-thirds of applicants to osteopathic programs also applied to allopathic programs; however, only one-seventh of allopathic program applicants also applied to osteopathic programs. Notably, as many as 72% of first-time applicants to offshore medical schools did not apply or had not ever applied to US allopathic or osteopathic programs. Ninety percent of all first-time applicants had applied to a US allopathic program.[98] There are currently no more recent data comparing applicant characteristics to offshore medical schools versus US allopathic and osteopathic programs. Research efforts have focused on comparing student performance with USMLE first time pass rates ranging from 19.4% to 84.4%, depending on country of medical school.[99] St. George's University, an offshore medical school located in the Caribbean, is certified by the Educational Commission for Foreign Medical Graduates and reports the average GPA and MCAT scores of their classes along with their admissions criteria. The variation in stent performance is also seen in match rates. St.

**Table 2**
**Matriculant data from 2018-2019 based on school type[100,103,104]**

|  | US Allopathic | US Osteopathic | St Georges University |
|---|---|---|---|
| Undergraduate GPA | 3.72 | 3.54 | 3.3 |
| Science GPA | 3.65 | 3.43 | 3.1 |
| Nonscience GPA | 3.8 | 3.65 | (Not provided) |
| MCAT overall | 511.2 | 503.83 | 497 |
| CPBS | 127.7 | 125.79 | 124 |
| CARS | 127.1 | 125.36 | 124 |
| BBLS | 128 | 126.16 | 124 |
| PSBB | 128.3 | 126.52 | 125 |
| Total women | 11,160 | 4118 | 3110 |
| Total men | 10,454 | 4317 | 3236 |

*Abbreviations:* BBLS, Biological and Biochemical Foundations of Living Systems; CARS, Critical Analysis and Reasoning Skills; CPBS, Chemical and Physical Foundations of Biological Systems; MCAT, Medical College Admission Test; PSBB, Psychological; Social, and Biological Foundations of Behavior.

George's boasts a 93% residency match rate, including international students who do not intend to pursue residency or practice in the United States after graduation.[100] For comparison, US allopathic programs had an overall 93% match rate, osteopathic programs a 91% match rate, and all offshore medical schools had an overall 61% match rate (**Table 2**).[101]

## ENROLLMENT MANAGEMENT MODELS

Although medical educators seem to believe admission to medical school should be governed, at least in part, by human judgment, there has been no systematic presentation of evidence suggesting it improves selection.[75] A meta-analyses of more than 150 studies demonstrate that mechanical/formula-based selection decisions actually produce better results than decisions made with holistic/clinical methods involving human judgment.[75] The use of holistic review as a method of incorporating human judgment is not a valid alternative to mechanical/statistical approaches; the evidence indicates clearly that mechanistic methods are more predictive, reliable, cost efficient, and transparent.[75] In another example, the enrollment predictions using the enrollment management model were at least as accurate as the expert human estimates. This information can be readily exported for a real-time dashboard system to drive recruitment behaviors.[102]

## SUMMARY

Moving beyond the standardized MCAT and GPA to select the best students for medical school admission is challenging. LORS, personal statements, and secondary applications essays continue to be used uniformly in medical student applications and selection despite questionable data validity. Although most medical schools tout holistic application reviews with a focus on the mission of the school, little evidence exists that this process is actually happening. Additionally, progress to improve access to URM has been slow, and additional efforts are needed to increase diversity in medical schools. Interviews for medical school acceptance are rapidly changing in this era of coronavirus disease 2019, with an increased emphasis on virtual interviewing. Increasing data support the use of MMIs and structured interviews over unstructured one-on-one interviews. Evidence is also increasing for the role of enrollment management models in the selection of medical students. Additional research is needed in the realm of artificial intelligence applicability in medical student selection.

## REFERENCES

1. Graduation Rates and Attrition Rates of U.S. Medical Students. Association of American Medical Colleges Student Records System. 2020. Available at: https://www.aamc.org/media/48526/download. Accessed November 15, 2020.

2. 2019 Performance Data. United States Medical Licensing Examination. Available at: https://www.usmle.org/performance-data/default.aspx#2019_overview. Accessed November 15, 2020.

3. Charting outcomes in the Match: senior students of U.S. MD medical schools. National Resident Matching Program. 2020. Available at: https://mk0nrmp3oyqui6wqfm.kinstacdn.com/wp-content/uploads/2020/07/Charting-Outcomes-in-the-Match-2020_MD-Senior_final.pdf. Accessed November 15, 2020.

4. Johnson DG. The AAMC study of medical student attrition: overview and major findings. J Med Educ 1965;40(10):913–20.

5. O'Neill LD, Wallstedt B, Eika B, et al. Factors associated with dropout in medical education: a literature review. Med Educ 2011;45(5):440–54.

6. Medical School Graduation and Attrition Rates. Association of American Medical Colleges. 2007. Available at: https://www.aamc.org/system/files/reports/1/aibvol7no2.pdf. Accessed November 15, 2020.

7. Medical Students' socioeconomic background and their completion of the first two years of medical school. Association of American Medical Colleges. 2010. Available at: https://www.aamc.org/system/files/reports/1/aibvol9_no11.pdf. Accessed November 15, 2020.

8. Applying to medical school with AMCAS. Association of American Medical Colleges. Available at: https://students-residents.aamc.org/applying-medical-school/applying-medical-school-process/applying-medical-school-amcas/. Accessed November 15, 2020.

9. Applicants, first-time applicants, and repeat applicants to U.S. medical schools, 1980-1981 through 2020-2021. Association of American Medical Colleges. 2020. Available at: https://www.aamc.org/media/9581/download. Accessed November 15, 2020.

10. Applicants, matriculants, enrollment, and graduates of U.S. medical schools, 2011-2012 through 2020-2021. Association of American Medical Colleges. 2020. Available at: https://www.aamc.org/media/37816/download. Accessed November 15, 2020.

11. Age of applicants to U.S. medical schools at anticipated matriculation by sex and race/ethnicity, 2014-2015 through 2017-2018. Association of American Medical Colleges. 2017. Available at: https://www.aamc.org/system/files/d/1/321468-factstablea6.pdf. Accessed November 15, 2020.

12. Applicants to U.S. medical schools by sex, 1980-1981 through 2020-2021. Association of American Medical Colleges. 2020. https://www.aamc.org/media/9586/download. Accessed November 15, 2020.

13. Cooper RA. Impact of trends in primary, secondary, and postsecondary education on applications to medical school. II: considerations of race, ethnicity, and income. Acad Med 2003;78(9):864–76.

14. Applicants to U.S. Medical Schools by Selected Combinations of Race/Ethnicity and Sex, 2017-20189 through 2020-2021. Association of American Medical Colleges. 2020. Available at: https://www.aamc.org/media/6026/download. Accessed November 15, 2020.

15. Capers Q, McDougle L, Clinchot DM. Strategies for achieving diversity through medical school admissions. J Health Care Poor Underserved 2018;29(1):9–18.

16. Thomas B, Manusov EG, Wang A, et al. Contributors of black men's success in admission to and graduation from medical school. Acad Med 2011;86(7): 892–900.

17. Stegers-Jager KM, Steyerberg EW, Lucieer SM, et al. Ethnic and social disparities in performance on medical school selection criteria. Med Educ 2015;49(1): 124–33.

18. Alexander C, Chen E, Grumbach K. How leaky is the health career pipeline? Minority student achievement in college gateway courses. Acad Med 2009;84(6): 797–802.

19. O'Neill L, Vonsild MC, Wallstedt B, et al. Admission criteria and diversity in medical school. Med Educ 2013;47(6):557–61.

20. Simmenroth-Nayda A, Görlich Y. Medical school admission test: advantages for students whose parents are medical doctors? BMC Med Educ 2015;15:81.

21. Wright B, Woloschuk W. Have rural background students been disadvantaged by the medical school admission process? Med Educ 2008;42(5):476–9.

22. Hutten-Czapski P, Pitblado R, Rourke J. Who gets into medical school? Comparison of students from rural and urban backgrounds. Can Fam Physician 2005; 51(9):1240–1.

23. MCAT and GPAs for Applicants and Matriculants to U.S. Medical Schools, 2017-2018 through 2020-2021. Association of American Medical Colleges. 2020. Available at: https://www.aamc.org/media/6056/download.

24. Gay SE, Santen SA, Mangrulkar RS, et al. The influence of MCAT and GPA preadmission academic metrics on interview scores. Adv Health Sci Educ Theory Pract 2018;23(1):151–8.

25. Agahi F, Speicher MR, Cisek G. Association between undergraduate performance predictors and academic and clinical performance of osteopathic medical students. J Am Osteopath Assoc 2018;118(2):106–14.

26. Lucchese M, Enders J, Burrone MS, et al. A study of success predictors in the entrance examination to the school medicine (2006-2008). Rev Fac Cien Med Univ Nac Cordoba 2010;67(1):50–5.

27. Yoho RM, Antonopoulos K, Vardaxis V. Undergraduate GPAs, MCAT scores, and academic performance the first 2 years in podiatric medical school at Des Moines University. J Am Podiatr Med Assoc 2012;102(6):446–50.

28. Poole P, Shulruf B, Rudland J, et al. Comparison of UMAT scores and GPA in prediction of performance in medical school: a national study. Med Educ 2012;46(2):163–71.

29. Luqman M. Relationship of academic success of medical students with motivation and pre-admission grades. J Coll Physicians Surg Pak 2013;23(1):31–6.

30. Salem RO, Al-Mously N, AlFadil S, et al. Pre-admission criteria and pre-clinical achievement: can they predict medical students performance in the clinical phase? Med Teach 2016;38(Suppl 1):S26–30.

31. Dixon D. Prediction of osteopathic medical school performance on the basis of MCAT score, GPA, sex, undergraduate major, and undergraduate institution. J Am Osteopath Assoc 2012;112(4):175–81.

32. Admissions Requirements. Association of American Medical Colleges. 2020. Available at: https://students-residents.aamc.org/applying-medical-school/applying-medical-school-process/medical-school-admission-requirements/admission-requirements/.

33. MCAT and GPAs for Applicants and Matriculants to U.S. Medical Schools by Primary Undergraduate Major, 2020-2021. Association of American Medical Colleges. 2020. https://www.aamc.org/media/6056/download.

34. Ellaway RH, Bates A, Girard S, et al. Exploring the consequences of combining medical students with and without a background in biomedical sciences. Med Educ 2014;48(7):674–86.

35. Houston M, Osborne M, Rimmer R. Private schooling and admission to medicine: a case study using matched samples and causal mediation analysis. BMC Med Educ 2015;15:136.

36. Gasman M, Smith T, Ye C, et al. HBCUs and the production of doctors. AIMS Public Health 2017;4(6):579–89.

37. Stratton TD, Elam CL, McGrath MG. A liberal arts education as preparation for medical school: how is it valued? How do graduates perform? Acad Med 2003;78(10 Suppl):S59–61.

38. Wilson I, Griffin B, Lampe L, et al. Variation in personality traits of medical students between schools of medicine. Med Teach 2013;35(11):944–8.

39. Andriole DA, Jeffe DB. Characteristics of medical school matriculants who participated in postbaccalaureate premedical programs. Acad Med 2011;86(2):201–10.

40. Grumbach K. Commentary: adopting postbaccalaureate premedical programs to enhance physician workforce diversity. Acad Med 2011;86(2):154–7.

41. Silver B, Hodgson CS. Evaluating GPAs and MCAT scores as predictors of NBME I and clerkship performances based on students' data from one undergraduate institution. Acad Med 1997;72(5):394–6.

42. Gauer JL, Wolff JM, Jackson JB. Do MCAT scores predict USMLE scores? An analysis on 5 years of medical student data. Med Educ Online 2016;21:31795.

43. Donnon T, Paolucci EO, Violato C. The predictive validity of the MCAT for medical school performance and medical board licensing examinations: a meta-analysis of the published research. Acad Med 2007;82(1):100–6.

44. Julian ER. Validity of the Medical College Admission Test for predicting medical school performance. Acad Med 2005;80(10):910–7.

45. Dunleavy DM, Kroopnick MH, Dowd KW, et al. The predictive validity of the MCAT exam in relation to academic performance through medical school: a national cohort study of 2001-2004 matriculants. Acad Med 2013;88(5):666–71.

46. Winegarden B, Glaser D, Schwartz A, et al. MCAT Verbal Reasoning score: less predictive of medical school performance for English language learners. Med Educ 2012;46(9):878–86.

47. Searcy CA, Dowd KW, Hughes MG, et al. Association of MCAT scores obtained with standard vs extra administration time with medical school admission, medical student performance, and time to graduation. JAMA 2015;313(22):2253–62.

48. Dixon D. Comparison of COMLEX-USA scores, medical school performance, and preadmission variables between women and men. J Am Osteopath Assoc 2015;115(4):222–5.

49. Terregino CA, Saguil A, Price-Johnson T, et al. The diversity and success of medical school applicants with scores in the middle third of the MCAT score scale. Acad Med 2020;95(3):344–50.
50. Khan JS, Tabasum S, Mukhtar O. Comparison of pre-medical academic achievement, entrance test and aptitude test scores in admission selection process. J Pak Med Assoc 2013;63(5):552–7.
51. Shipley TW, Phu N, Etters AM, et al. Comprehensive medical college admission test preparatory course as a strategy to encourage premedical students to pursue osteopathic medicine in rural areas. J Am Osteopath Assoc 2019;119(4): 243–9.
52. Griffin B, Auton J, Duvivier R, et al. Applicants to medical school: if at first they don't succeed, who tries again and are they successful? Adv Health Sci Educ Theory Pract 2019;24(1):33–43.
53. Grbic D, Brewer Roskovensky L. Which factors predict the likelihood of reapplying to medical school? An analysis by gender. Acad Med 2012;87(4):449–57.
54. Kim SH. Extracurricular activities of medical school applicants. Korean J Med Educ 2016;28(2):201–7.
55. Urlings-Strop LC, Themmen APN, Stegers-Jager KM. The relationship between extracurricular activities assessed during selection and during medical school and performance. Adv Health Sci Educ Theory Pract 2017;22(2):287–98.
56. Sparano DM, Shofer FS, Hollander JE. Participation in the academic associate program: effect on medical school admission rate. Acad Emerg Med 2004; 11(6):695–8.
57. Blue AV, Basco WT Jr, Geesey ME, et al. How does pre-admission community service compare with community service during medical school? Teach Learn Med 2005;17(4):316–21.
58. Fukawa-Connelly K, Tolen R, Lovold D. Crafting your personal statement. Association of American Medical Colleges. 2017. Available at: https://students-residents. aamc.org/choosing-medical-career/article/advisor-corner-crafting-your-personal-statement/. Accessed November 15, 2020.
59. Arbelaez C, Ganguli I. The personal statement for residency application: review and guidance. J Natl Med Assoc 2011;103(5):439–42.
60. Katzung KG, Ankel F, Clark M, et al. What do program directors look for in an applicant? J Emerg Med 2019;56(5):e95–101.
61. Elam CL, Stratton TD, Scott KL, et al. Review, deliberation, and voting: a study of selection decisions in a medical school admission committee. Teach Learn Med 2002;14(2):98–103.
62. Patterson F, Knight A, Dowell J, et al. How effective are selection methods in medical education? A systematic review. Med Educ 2016;50(1):36–60.
63. Lievens F. Diversity in medical school admission: insights from personnel recruitment and selection. Med Educ 2015;49(1):11–4.
64. Dong T, Kay A, Artino AR Jr, et al. Application essays and future performance in medical school: are they related? Teach Learn Med 2013;25(1):55–8.
65. Ghaffari Rafi A. Secondary medical school applications place an unfair financial burden on middle- and lower-income applicants. Acad Med 2017;92(6):728.
66. Matriculating Student Questionnaire, 2019 All Schools Summary Report. Association of American Medical Colleges. Available at: https://www.aamc.org/system/files/2019-12/2019%20MSQ%20All%20Schools%20Summary%20Report.pdf. Accessed November 15, 2020.
67. How Social Media Can Affect Your Application. Association of American Medical Colleges. Available at: https://students-residents.aamc.org/applying-medical-

school/article/how-social-media-can-affect-your-application/. Accessed November 15, 2020.

68. Witzburg RA, Sondheimer HM. Holistic review–shaping the medical profession one applicant at a time. N Engl J Med 2013;368(17):1565–7.

69. Ray R, Brown J. Reassessing student potential for medical school success: distance traveled, grit, and hardiness. Mil Med 2015;180(4 Suppl):138–41.

70. DeZee KJ, Magee CD, Rickards G, et al. What aspects of letters of recommendation predict performance in medical school? Findings from one institution. Acad Med 2014;89(10):1408–15.

71. Dirschl DR, Adams GL. Reliability in evaluating letters of recommendation. Acad Med 2000;75(10):1029.

72. Albanese MA, Snow MH, Skochelak SE, et al. Assessing personal qualities in medical school admissions. Acad Med 2003;78(3):313–21.

73. Siu E, Reiter HI. Overview: what's worked and what hasn't as a guide towards predictive admissions tool development. Adv Health Sci Educ Theory Pract 2009;14(5):759–75.

74. Holistic Review in Medical School Admissions. Association of American Medical Colleges. 2020. Available at: https://students-residents.aamc.org/choosing-medical-career/article/holistic-review-medical-school-admissions/. Accessed November 15, 2020.

75. Kreiter C, O'Shea M, Bruen C, et al. A meta-analytic perspective on the valid use of subjective human judgement to make medical school admission decisions. Med Educ Online 2018;23(1):1522225.

76. Eva KW, Reiter HI, Rosenfeld J, et al. The ability of the multiple mini-interview to predict preclerkship performance in medical school. Acad Med 2004;79(10 Suppl):S40–2.

77. Reiter HI, Eva KW, Rosenfeld J, et al. Multiple mini-interviews predict clerkship and licensing examination performance. Med Educ 2007;41(4):378–84.

78. Griffin BN, Wilson IG. Interviewer bias in medical student selection. Med J Aust 2010;193(6):343–6.

79. Eva KW, Macala C, Fleming B. Twelve tips for constructing a multiple mini-interview. Med Teach 2019;41(5):510–6.

80. Kelly ME, Patterson F, O'Flynn S, et al. A systematic review of stakeholder views of selection methods for medical schools admission. BMC Med Educ 2018; 18(1):139.

81. Razack S, Hodges B, Steinert Y, et al. Seeking inclusion in an exclusive process: discourses of medical school student selection. Med Educ 2015;49(1):36–47.

82. Raghavan M, Burnett M, Martin BD, et al. Utility of a writing station in the multiple mini-interview. J Vet Med Educ 2013;40(2):177–83.

83. Ali S, Sadiq Hashmi MS, Umair M, et al. Multiple mini-interviews: current perspectives on utility and limitations. Adv Med Educ Pract 2019;10:1031–8.

84. Reiter HI, Lockyer J, Ziola B, et al. Should efforts in favor of medical student diversity be focused during admissions or farther upstream? Acad Med 2012; 87(4):443–8.

85. Terregino CA, McConnell M, Reiter HI. The effect of differential weighting of academics, experiences, and competencies measured by multiple mini interview (MMI) on race and ethnicity of cohorts accepted to one medical school. Acad Med 2015;90(12):1651–7.

86. About CASPer. Computer-based assessment for sampling personal characteristics 2020.

87. Juster FR, Baum RC, Zou C, et al. Addressing the diversity-validity dilemma using situational judgment tests. Acad Med 2019;94(8):1197–203.
88. O'Connell RL, Kemp MT, Alam HB. The potential impact of COVID-19 on the medical school application. J Med Educ Curric Dev 2020;7. 2382120520940666.
89. Sims SM, Lynch JW. Medical educational culture: introducing patients to applicants as part of the medical school interview: feasibility and initial impact show and tell. Med Educ Online 2016;21:31760.
90. Talmor AG, Falk A, Almog Y. A new admission method may select applicants with a distinct personality profile. Med Teach 2017;39(6):646–52.
91. Kulasegaram K, Reiter HI, Wiesner W, et al. Non-association between Neo-5 personality tests and multiple mini-interview. Adv Health Sci Educ Theory Pract 2010;15(3):415–23.
92. Cook CJ, Cook CE, Hilton TN. Does emotional intelligence influence success during medical school admissions and program matriculation? A systematic review. J Educ Eval Health Prof 2016;13:40.
93. Hanson MD, Eva KW. A reflection upon the impact of early 21st-century technological innovations on medical school admissions. Acad Med 2019;94(5):640–4.
94. Daboub JA, Bergemann AD, Smith SR. Rethinking an admissions program to align with the mission of an innovative medical school. Med Sci Educ 2020;1–5. https://doi.org/10.1007/s40670-020-01084-y.
95. Ballejos MP, Oglesbee S, Hettema J, et al. An equivalence study of interview platform: does videoconference technology impact medical school acceptance rates of different groups? Adv Health Sci Educ Theory Pract 2018;23(3):601–10.
96. The AAMC video interview tool for admissions: essentials for the 2021 application cycle. Association of American Medical Colleges. 2020. Available at: https://aamc-orange.global.ssl.fastly.net/production/media/filer_public/37/b7/37b757f1-0363-4880-952c-e44e84ba0380/vita_essentials_-_web_final_7162020.pdf.
97. Bibler Zaidi NL, Santen SA, Purkiss JA, et al. A hybrid interview model for medical school interviews: combining traditional and multisampling formats. Acad Med 2016;91(11):1526–9.
98. Jolly P, Garrison G, Boulet JR, et al. Three pathways to a physician career: applicants to U.S. MD and DO schools and U.S. Citizen applicants to international medical schools. Acad Med 2008;83(12):1125–31.
99. van Zanten M, Boulet JR. Medical education in the Caribbean: a longitudinal study of United States Medical Licensing Examination performance, 2000-2009. Acad Med 2011;86(2):231–8.
100. Enrollment and Demographics. St. George's University. 2019. Available at: https://www.sgu.edu/enrollment-and-demographics-school-of-medicine/. Accessed November 15, 2020.
101. Medical students match in record numbers, celebrate virtually. American Medical Association. 2020. Available at: https://www.ama-assn.org/residents-students/match/medical-students-match-record-numbers-celebrate-virtually. Accessed November 15, 2020.
102. Burkhardt JC, DesJardins SL, Teener CA, et al. Predicting medical school enrollment behavior: comparing an enrollment management model to expert human judgment. Acad Med 2018;93(11S Association of American Medical Colleges Learn Serve Lead: Proceedings of the 57th Annual Research in Medical Education Sessions):S68–73. https://doi.org/10.1097/acm.0000000000002374.
103. MCAT Scores and GPAs for Applicants to U.S. Medical Schools by Sex, 2017-2018 through 2020-2021. Association of American Medical Colleges. 2020.

Available at: https://www.aamc.org/media/6081/download. Accessed November 15, 2020.

104. AACOMAS Applicant and Matriculant Profile Summary Report. American Association of Colleges of Osteopathic Medicine. 2018. Available at: https://www.aacom.org/docs/default-source/data-and-trends/2018-aacomas-applicant-matriculant-profile-summary-report.pdf. Accessed November 15, 2020.

# Attracting the Best Students to a Surgical Career

Cameron St. Hilaire, MD, Tatyana Kopilova, MD, Jeffrey M. Gauvin, MD, MS*

## KEYWORDS

- Medical students • Surgical education • Career choice • Surgeon workforce
- Implicit bias

## KEY POINTS

- There is a predicted shortage of surgeons in the future workforce. This is already occurring in rural areas and is expected to get much worse.
- US allopathic medical school graduates have been losing interest in surgery for the past 40 years, and this disturbing trend continues today; the residency match remains unaffected because of foreign and osteopathic applicants.
- Negative myths with regard to surgeon training, lifestyle, and personality persist among medical students and serve as a deterrent to choosing a surgical career.
- Proven strategies for making surgery more attractive to students are not always used and can be as simple as getting early exposure to students well before their clinical rotations.

## INTRODUCTION

In the 2001 to 2002 National Resident Matching Program (NRMP), there were an unexpected large number of unfilled, general surgery positions that left 68 programs without a full complement.[1] This finding came to many as a great surprise, as the number of applicants had always outnumbered the available positions, and US surgery programs had a long tradition of always filling. Because the number of applicants had always outnumbered the available positions, few took notice of a long trend that had been occurring among US allopathic medical students. The interest in general surgery by US medical school graduates had been decreasing for decades before the 2001 to 2002 match. More surprising, this trend continues today.

Immediately following that disastrous match, things appeared to have corrected. The subsequent NRMP match rates for surgery stabilized at nearly 100%, where they remain today. What is likely missed by many is that, despite the corrected match rates, interest in general surgery by US allopathic medical school graduates continues to decrease as it has done for the past 4 decades.

Department of Surgical Education, 400 West Pueblo Street, Santa Barbara, CA 93105, USA
* Corresponding author.
E-mail address: jgauvin@sbch.org

Surg Clin N Am 101 (2021) 653–665
https://doi.org/10.1016/j.suc.2021.05.011
0039-6109/21/© 2021 Elsevier Inc. All rights reserved.

Many believe the implementation of the 80-hour workweek along with other work hour restrictions that followed remedied the declining interest of US medical graduates, but this is simply not true. Although surgery match rates immediately rebounded and remain near 100%, the interest in general surgery by US medical school graduates has significantly decreased. The percentage of US seniors matching into general surgery dropped from 12% in 1980 to 5.8% in 2011.[1] The spots not filled by American allopathic seniors have gone to osteopathic and international graduates.

The problem of declining medical student interest in surgical careers is not unique to the United States. The Canadian Resident Matching Service saw a reduction of graduating medical students ranking surgical specialties as their first choice from 24% in 1998 to 17.2% in 2016. During this same period, there was an increase in the proportion of Canadian medical students opting for "controllable lifestyle" specialties, such as radiology, anesthesiology, and emergency medicine.[2–4]

What makes this trend so alarming is the predicted shortage of general surgeons. Because of a growing and aging US population, the future of the general surgery workforce will likely be insufficient to serve the needs of the population. There will be a 15% to 21% shortage in the number of general surgeons by the year 2050.[5] This pending problem will be even worse in rural areas where they are already suffering from a lack of surgeons.

As we look to recruit the best students into our profession, it is worthwhile to take a brief look at our interesting and often overlooked history of training doctors. When it came to training its students, the medical profession did not always get it right.

### Historical Side Note

Although physicians may be held in high regard in today's society, that was not always the case. Not many medical professionals today are aware of the controversial start that medical education had in this and other counties. Few know that one of the first large-scale riots that occurred in the United States was a result of medical education gone wrong. In the eighteenth century, grave robbing was so common that family members of the recently deceased would often spend many days at the graveside to the deter "resurrectionists," whose profession it was to rob the bodies of the recently buried and sell them to medical schools. In 1788, John Hicks was a medical student at Columbia College, New York's only medical school. He was dissecting the arm of a cadaver when some children caught his attention out of a window. It has been said that Hicks waved the arm at the group of children and yelled "this is your mother's arm! I just dug it up." The mother of one of the children had just died. The child ran home and told his grieving father what happened. After exhuming his wife's coffin to find it empty, the enraged father gathered friends and neighbors and a mob soon formed.

Over several days, the mob swelled to an estimated 5000. Doctors and medical students fled, and hospital apartments and anatomy laboratories were destroyed. Eventually, the mayor and sheriff escorted some of the doctors and students to jail in an effort to protect them. After Columbia alumnus, Alexander Hamilton, was unable to quell the mob, the governor of New York called out the militia in an effort to bring peace. John Jay (who later became the first Chief Justice of the Supreme Court) was struck in the head with a rock, and Revolutionary War hero, General Baron von Steuben, was hit with a brick. After this, despite orders to not fire their muskets, the militia opened fire on the crowd. At least 3 rioters and 3 militia were killed with final casualty estimates as high as 20. This event would be become known as the "Doctor's Riot."[6]

We have certainly come a long way in the past 240 years. However, given the predicted surgeon shortage and the sustained decreasing interest in surgery by medical students, it is paramount that we understand what factors currently drive this generation of medical students to choose a specialty if we hope to mitigate this shortage and create more general surgery graduates. We simply must understand how to attract more and better students to the field.

It is hoped that surgical educators can evoke some positive changes. Some of these factors may prove to be low-hanging fruit that can be easily changed, while others may prove harder to reach.

## DISCUSSION

All US medical students spend between 4 and 12 weeks on surgery rotations. It follows that many opportunities to influence students in a positive way toward surgery during these rotations must exist. In addition, there are substantial data to suggest that involvement with medical students much earlier in medical school may have significant benefits. A 2005 survey found that 45% of first-year medical students were interested in a surgical career, yet only 7% of graduating students matched into surgical residencies.[7] Student interest in surgery as a career is highest in the first year of medical school and decreases by 5% in each subsequent year.[8] These data should prompt us to get involved with medical students as early as possible and understand what factors are in play that make surgery become so unpopular. We focus our discussion on examining what we know and what we might be able to do about reversing this trend.

### Preclinical Education

Multiple studies have shown exposure to surgery before the clinical rotations has a positive influence on medical student interest in surgery.[9–18] Following the exposure, students had greater understanding that surgery can still allow for work-life balance and evoke meaningful change in patients' lives. Development of formal preclinical surgical exposure programs also has a positive effect on students' attitudes toward the surgical culture. In addition, they enhance confidence in the operating room (OR).[19]

Kassam and colleagues[8] found students identifying a mentor *before* the start of their surgery clerkship resulted in higher interest after the rotation. Lazow and colleagues[19] also found a similar trend when preclinical students participated in a 1-month, hands-on surgery program. Of the program participants, 71.4% went on to match into surgical fields compared with 21.7% of nonparticipants.

### Mentorship

Surgical mentors can have a strong influence on a medical student's career choice. In fact, 98% of students expressing an interest in surgery identified a positive influence at some stage of their training.[20] According to a review by Peel and colleagues,[21] 26 studies reported the presence of a surgical role model to be a significant positive influence on surgical career decision making. Students had a significantly greater interest in surgery when partnered with a mentor, whereas the absence of such a mentor was a deterrent.

Cochran and colleagues[22] reported the identification of a surgical mentor to be an important factor correlating with medical students' decision to pursue surgery compared with those planning a nonsurgical career. Multiple studies have shown that medical students interested in surgery and general surgery residency applicants emphasized the positive effect of a faculty role model more so than students interested in other specialties.[23,24] In fact, multiple studies have demonstrated that a mentorship-based, preclinical, surgical elective significantly improved junior medical student confidence and increased the likelihood that those students would be interested in a surgical career.[25,26]

Cook and colleagues[27] revealed that students who rotated at the nonmetropolitan center with a one-on-one clerkship experience with faculty mentors had a drastically increased interest in surgery compared with those who completed a more "classic" surgery rotation in a metropolitan university teaching hospital setting.

There is also a positive association between exposure to surgical residents and interest in a surgical career. It is thought that resident exposure is particularly effective because of the extent to which students and residents interact; surgical residents can be outstanding mentors and role models for our medical students and positively influence students to pursue surgery.[28,29] Furthermore, students exposed to the highest rated surgical residents were even more likely to pursue surgical residency training compared with those students who worked with less effective residents.[30]

A study by Pointer and colleagues[31] highlights the importance of the mentorship/role model experience. In their survey, the most important factors cited for choosing general surgery as a career were perceived career enjoyment of residents and faculty, resident/faculty relationships, and mentorship. Surgery residents were viewed as role models by 72%, and faculty were viewed as role models by 77%. This study demonstrated almost half of those choosing a surgical career did so as a direct result of the core rotation experience. The authors believe that structuring the medical student experience to optimize the interaction of students, residents, and faculty produces a positive environment, encouraging students to choose a general surgery career.

### Clerkship Experience

Although exposure to surgeons and surgical mentors at all levels of medical school can be important, the surgery clerkship experience can have the greatest influence. There have been numerous surveys demonstrating the impact the surgery clerkship plays in the decision to pursue a career in surgery. Students who had a positive experience in their surgery clerkship had a significantly higher preference toward general surgery.[32] In a large 2018 review, Peel and colleagues[21] found a total of 21 studies that assessed the association of clinical exposure and medical student interest in surgery.[21] Of these, 11 showed that clinical exposure improved both surgical knowledge and interest in surgery as a career. They found 6 studies that looked at the effect of the surgical clerkship on student perceptions. Four of these showed an increase in student's interest in surgical topics and showed students the potential for work-life balance in surgeon's lives, thus increasing interest in surgery careers.

Ko and colleagues[33] found that a strong predictor for a student entering general surgery was satisfaction with the quality of attending teaching. They found that certain instructional choices made by faculty could significantly help promote student satisfaction; for instance, allowing a student to actively participate in an operation (ie, suturing, cutting) and doing fewer passive things like retracting and simply observing. Another study showed that students who were engaged in the OR were 5 to 7 times as likely to be interested in surgery; students who sutured in the OR were 4.8 times more likely to be interested in surgery; and students who drove the camera during a laparoscopic case were 7.2 times more likely.[34] In a recent large review, Marshall and colleagues[35] found that a positive experience during surgical rotations was associated with a higher interest in a career in surgery and confirmed that active involvement in the OR was important. Marshall and colleagues35 also found that a welcoming environment in the OR for medical students was important and advises helping students avoid presyncopal and syncopal episodes in the operating theater may also help to improve medical student experience.

In addition, the type and length of the surgical clerkship can have a significant effect. Clerkships at nontraditional community-based hospitals have been found to be a positive experience for medical students. Clerkship rotations at a community hospital result in medical students feeling reassured that surgeons can maintain work-life balance.[26,27] Similarly, apprenticeship models not only improved the clerkship experience but also improved medical students' perception of surgeons.[36] Longer-length clerkships may also be better at increasing surgery clerkship satisfaction and interest; shorter clerkships may have an adverse effect.[33]

Four studies assessed the effect of surgical simulation training on the clerkship experience; all were found to improve the experience, and 2 demonstrated improved interest in surgery.[37–40]

Modifiable clerkship factors:
- Make students feel welcome in the OR
- Assure active involvement in operations
- Clearly define the student's role
- Assure effective role modeling and assign a mentor
- Encourage student and resident interactions
- Allow students to participate in simulation when available
- Consider lengthening the clerkship duration

### Lifestyle

Many studies demonstrate the perceived lifestyle of surgical trainees and practicing surgeons is a major deterrent from a career in surgery.[7,41–45] In an extensive review that looked at multiple factors that affected medical student career choice, surgical lifestyle and its impact were the most heavily studied.[21] Twenty-two studies that were reviewed explicitly commented on the weight that students place on the duration of training and work-life balance when choosing their career. Most medical students saw the career-focused surgical lifestyle as their primary deterrent from surgical specialties. Students that were already interested in surgery considered lifestyle less important when deciding on a career.

The importance of lifestyle is not confined to North America. A survey about student perceptions of a general surgery career was distributed to 9 medical schools in 8 countries. The most important reason for not choosing general surgery was because of perceptions of an unpleasant lifestyle. The negative influence of "lifestyle" persisted across all countries, both sexes, and all levels of socioeconomic development.[46] The investigators concluded the negative influence of lifestyle is the most important reason contemporary medical students from different parts of the world choose not to pursue general surgery. Strategies to counteract the perceived unfriendly nature of the lifestyle are essential to increase the interest of contemporary medical students toward general surgery.

Much of the data collected in many of these reviews is outdated as is the current thinking of current medical students regarding the surgical life. Simply informing students of current changes to our profession may go a long way in promoting more interest in our profession. The clerkship experience can improve interest in surgical careers by simply dispelling the myth that surgery precludes work-life balance.[26,47,48] For instance, students were unaware of the Acute Care Surgery model, even after completion of their clerkship. Their interest increased once the lifestyle and practice advantages of this subspecialty were explained to them.[49]

### Personality Type

Multiple studies have shown an association of certain personality traits that predispose an individual to an interest in surgery.[50–55] These individuals are significantly more extroverted and conscientious than the general population as well as significantly less impulsive. Other studies suggested that students who valued prestige, financial gain, and academic ambition more frequently pursue careers in surgery.[56–60]

A European study looked at personality traits and found there were reproducible tendencies of surgeons to score higher in extraversion, openness to experience, and emotional stability compared with internal medicine physicians. This finding held true across board-certified, resident, and medical student cohorts.[55,61] Moreover, out of all surgical trainees, the high performing ones seem to score higher in extraversion, conscientiousness, and emotional stability categories when compared with non-high-performing residents based on residency performance and standardized test scores.[62]

### Implicit Bias and Misinformation

In an excellent review article that examined factors affecting medical student career decisions, Schmidt and colleagues[63] highlight that a major uphill battle in the recruitment of medical students to general surgery is the stereotype of surgeons perceived by medical students at all levels. One of these studies by Kozar and colleagues[64] found that negative perceptions by medical students toward surgery came from a variety of sources, such as fellow classmates, preceptors, and media, and could negatively impact their decision to choose a surgical career. Hill and colleagues[42] identified several areas where the stereotypes of surgery (competitive, masculine, and requiring sacrifice) and surgeons (self-confident and intimidating) limited medical student's interest in surgery. In addition, Sanfey and colleagues[43] found 70% of medical students believed surgeons do not lead well-balanced lives and saw this as a deterrent to pursuing a surgical career. Conversely, when students had encounters with surgeons who discussed their professional and personal lives, it favorably influenced the perception of medical students toward a surgical career.[22]

### Gender

A position statement from the Association of Women Surgeons expressed ongoing concern regarding gender bias and gender discrimination that has deterred female interest in surgery.[65] Gender discrimination is reported across all medical specialties, and is not unique to surgery; however, the perception of gender bias is frequently reported during surgical experiences and has been shown to decrease interest in the pursuit of further surgical training.[66–78] Significantly fewer female than male medical students considered surgical careers and ranked surgical residencies.[71,79]

Many studies report that a significant portion of female medical students experience gender discrimination and that this influences their career decisions.[66,68–71,79–81] The lack of female role models is also frequently reported as a reason for reduced interest in surgery among female students. It has been shown that female students are significantly more likely to enter specialties with a higher proportion of women.[41,82]

Peel and colleagues[21] propose that historical and ongoing gender discrimination has resulted in underrepresentation of women in surgery, especially in leadership roles and academia.[21] This underrepresentation may be perceived as a "glass ceiling" hindering career development of women in surgery, thereby discouraging more women from considering careers in surgery. As an effort has been made to improve representation of women in surgery, the authors recommend that ongoing effort be made to demonstrate inclusion and equal opportunity within surgery.

Although both men and women consider practice lifestyle in choosing their medical careers, Wendel and colleagues[41] found that fewer women than men considered practice lifestyle when choosing their career, but men had more interest in pursuing surgery after completion of their clerkship. In addition, female students were more likely to state that gender discrimination was a deterrent. Women also preferred residency programs where parental leave and on-site childcare were available. Female students are more easily deterred by the "surgical personality."[82]

## SUMMARY

The general surgery match has largely been unaffected by the declining interest of US allopathic medical students in surgery. So why does it matter if these spots are now being filled with osteopathic students and foreign graduates? It may not, as some of the best residents and surgeons come from this pool of applicants (Gauvin, personal observation). However, wanting to avoid another crisis, like the 2001 to 2002 match, might prove to be enough motivation. By simply increasing the overall quality of the applicant pool, program directors may be able to build stronger programs that can soon expand in order to mitigate the pending surgeon shortage.

Certain nonmodifiable features of surgical life cannot be changed, and these will continue to deter students from surgery. However, there is much that can be done by surgeons and educators, at all levels of training that have proven effective to increase interest in surgery.

Preclinical Years
- Become involved early in medical student education.
- Participate in surgery interest groups.
- In all encounters, make an effort to dispel the myths of the "surgeon personality." Be kind and patient teachers and better role models.
- Ensure work-life balance is possible and talk of your life outside of work.
Modifiable clerkship factors:
- Make students feel welcome in the OR, assure active involvement in operations, and clearly define their role.
- Assign a mentor and assure effective role modeling.
- Make life balance an additional learning objective in the surgical clerkship.
- Encourage resident and student interactions.
- Allow students to participate in simulation training.
- Consider setting aside time each week for "student walk rounds." Use the opportunity to dispel the myth of the surgeon as a cold, unfeeling technician and let students see the surgeon as a compassionate, caring physician and kind teacher.
Gender
- Be aware that gender bias is frequently reported during surgical experiences.
- A significant portion of female medical students experience gender discrimination, and this influences their career decisions.
- We must continue our efforts to change the ongoing gender discrimination that resulted in underrepresentation of women in surgery.
- Departments must work to recruit more women surgeons; a lack of female role models is frequently reported as a reason for reduced interest in surgery among female students

One last and perhaps controversial thought: maybe our medical schools are failing us. Acceptance to allopathic medical schools has become much more competitive over the last few decades with strong emphasis on grade point average (GPA) and sexy volunteer experiences. Perhaps the effort to recruit people who have the financial resources to add countless volunteer experiences, who research, and who take review courses and thus present a polished and well-financed curriculum vitae and high GPA may be misplaced. Other, less privileged students, who may be busy working to support themselves through school, may not be as readily admitted to our medical schools. The grit and distance traveled by this group of applicants might be just what has been missing in many of our medical students. Are we underestimating the importance of this work ethic? "Distance traveled" should be given more weight when measuring the mettle of our medical school applicants. Maybe recruiting more from this pool will again allow us to have classes full of hard-working, passionate students who understand that residency is a job, not a glorified class, and gladly welcome the rigors of a surgical career and not just settle for a "lifestyle profession."

Ours is indeed the greatest discipline within all of medicine. This statement has been told to the senior author of this work, most often not by surgeons or surgical residents, but by students who have chosen not to match in surgery. They regrettably opt for less-appealing careers based mostly on lifestyle concerns and the myth that being a good parent or spouse is not possible if one is also a surgeon.

Be upbeat and enthusiastic about our specialty, but be sure to let students see the richness of your life outside of surgery. Let them see you as an involved parent, Little League coach, and attentive spouse.

- There is a predicted future shortage of surgeons in the workforce. This is already occurring in rural areas and is expected to get worse.
- US allopathic medical school graduates have been losing interest in surgery for the past 40 years, and this disturbing trend continues.
- The match remains unaffected because of foreign graduates and osteopathic applicants.
- Negative myths regarding surgeon training, lifestyle, and personality persist among medical students and can be a powerful deterrent to a surgical career.
- Proven strategies for making surgery more attractive to students are not always used.
- Things as simple as getting early exposure to students well before their clinical rotations and talking about your life outside of work can have great effect.
- Perhaps we should encourage medical schools to lengthen the surgical clerkship.

## DISCLOSURE

The authors have nothing to disclose.

## REFERENCES

1. National Resident Matching Program. Report archives 2020. Available at: https://www.nrmp.org/report-archives/. Accessed 2020.
2. Pukite J, Pukite P. Modeling for reliability analysis - Markov modeling for reliability, maintainability, safety, and supportability analyses of complex systems. 1998.
3. Scott IM, Matejcek AN, Gowans MC, et al. Choosing a career in surgery: factors that influence Canadian medical students' interest in pursuing a surgical career. Can J Surg 2008;51(5):371-7.

4. Service CRM. Canadian residency matching service report. CaRMS. CaRMS Web site. Accessed2016.

5. Ellison EC, Pawlik TM, Way DP, et al. Ten-year reassessment of the shortage of general surgeons: increases in graduation numbers of general surgery residents are insufficient to meet the future demand for general surgeons. Surgery 2018; 164(4):726–32.

6. de Costa C, Miller F. American resurrection and the 1788 New York doctors' riot. Lancet 2011;377(9762):292–3.

7. Brundage SI, Lucci A, Miller CC, et al. Potential targets to encourage a surgical career. J Am Coll Surg 2005;200(6):946–53.

8. Kassam AF, Cortez AR, Winer LK, et al. The impact of medical student interest in surgery on clerkship performance and career choice. Am J Surg 2020;219(2): 359–65.

9. Zuckerman SL, Mistry AM, Hanif R, et al. Neurosurgery elective for preclinical medical students: early exposure and changing attitudes. World Neurosurg 2016;86:120–6.

10. Khatib M, Soukup B, Boughton O, et al. Plastic surgery undergraduate training: how a single local event can inspire and educate medical students. Ann Plast Surg 2015;75(2):208–12.

11. Davis CR, O'Donoghue JM, McPhail J, et al. How to improve plastic surgery knowledge, skills and career interest in undergraduates in one day. J Plast Reconstr Aesthet Surg 2010;63(10):1677–81.

12. Cloyd J, Holtzman D, O'Sullivan P, et al. Operating room assist: surgical mentorship and operating room experience for preclerkship medical students. J Surg Educ 2008;65(4):275–82.

13. Day KM, Schwartz TM, Rao V, et al. Medical student clerkship performance and career selection after a junior medical student surgical mentorship program. Am J Surg 2016;211(2):431–6.

14. Teo LL, Venkatesh SK, Goh PS, et al. A survey of local preclinical and clinical medical students' attitudes towards radiology. Ann Acad Med Singap 2010; 39(9):692–4.

15. Are C, Stoddard HA, Thompson JS, et al. The influence of surgical demonstrations during an anatomy course on the perceptions of first-year medical students toward surgeons and a surgical career. J Surg Educ 2010;67(5):320–4.

16. Gawad N, Moussa F, Christakis GT, et al. Planting the 'SEAD': early comprehensive exposure to surgery for medical students. J Surg Educ 2013;70(4):487–94.

17. George J, Combellack T, Lopez-Marco A, et al. Winning hearts and minds: inspiring medical students into cardiothoracic surgery through highly interactive workshops. J Surg Educ 2017;74(2):372–6.

18. Pulcrano ME, Malekzadeh S, Kumar A. The impact of gross anatomy laboratory on first year medical students' interest in a surgical career. Clin Anat 2016; 29(6):691–5.

19. Lazow SP, Venn RA, Lubor B, et al. The PreOp program: intensive preclinical surgical exposure is associated with increased medical student surgical interest and competency. J Surg Educ 2019;76(5):1278–85.

20. Ek EW, Ek ET, Mackay SD. Undergraduate experience of surgical teaching and its influence and its influence on career choice. ANZ J Surg 2005;75(8):713–8.

21. Peel JK, Schlachta CM, Alkhamesi NA. A systematic review of the factors affecting choice of surgery as a career. Can J Surg 2018;61(1):58–67.

22. Cochran A, Melby S, Neumayer LA. An Internet-based survey of factors influencing medical student selection of a general surgery career. Am J Surg 2005; 189(6):742–6.

23. Quillin RC 3rd, Pritts TA, Davis BR, et al. Surgeons underestimate their influence on medical students entering surgery. J Surg Res 2012;177(2):201–6.

24. Erzurum VZ, Obermeyer RJ, Fecher A, et al. What influences medical students' choice of surgical careers. Surgery 2000;128(2):253–6.

25. Drolet BC, Sangisetty S, Mulvaney PM, et al. A mentorship-based preclinical elective increases exposure, confidence, and interest in surgery. Am J Surg 2014;207(2):179–86.

26. Carter MB, Larson GM, Polk HC Jr. A brief private group practice rotation changes junior medical students' perception of the surgical lifestyle. Am J Surg 2005;189(4):458–61.

27. Cook MR, Yoon M, Hunter J, et al. A nonmetropolitan surgery clerkship increases interest in a surgical career. Am J Surg 2015;209(1):21–5.

28. Whittaker LD Jr, Estes NC, Ash J, et al. The value of resident teaching to improve student perceptions of surgery clerkships and surgical career choices. Am J Surg 2006;191(3):320–4.

29. Nguyen SQ, Divino CM. Surgical residents as medical student mentors. Am J Surg 2007;193(1):90–3.

30. Musunuru S, Lewis B, Rikkers LF, et al. Effective surgical residents strongly influence medical students to pursue surgical careers. J Am Coll Surg 2007;204(1): 164–7.

31. Pointer DT Jr, Freeman MD, Korndorffer JR Jr, et al. Choosing surgery: identifying factors leading to increased general surgery matriculation rate. Am Surg 2017; 83(3):290–5.

32. Al-Heeti KN, Nassar AK, Decorby K, et al. The effect of general surgery clerkship rotation on the attitude of medical students towards general surgery as a future career. J Surg Educ 2012;69(4):544–9.

33. Ko CY, Escarce JJ, Baker L, et al. Predictors for medical students entering a general surgery residency: national survey results. Surgery 2004;136(3):567–72.

34. Berman L, Rosenthal MS, Curry LA, et al. Attracting surgical clerks to surgical careers: role models, mentoring, and engagement in the operating room. J Am Coll Surg 2008;207(6):793–800, 800.e1-2.

35. Marshall DC, Salciccioli JD, Walton SJ, et al. Medical student experience in surgery influences their career choices: a systematic review of the literature. J Surg Educ 2015;72(3):438–45.

36. Reid CM, Kim DY, Mandel J, et al. Impact of a third-year surgical apprenticeship model: perceptions and attitudes compared with the traditional medical student clerkship experience. J Am Coll Surg 2014;218(5):1032–7.

37. Galiñanes EL, Shirshenkan JR, Doty J, et al. Standardized laparoscopic simulation positively affects a student's surgical experience. J Surg Educ 2013;70(4): 508–13.

38. Lee JT, Qiu M, Teshome M, et al. The utility of endovascular simulation to improve technical performance and stimulate continued interest of preclinical medical students in vascular surgery. J Surg Educ 2009;66(6):367–73.

39. Lee JT, Son JH, Chandra V, et al. Long-term impact of a preclinical endovascular skills course on medical student career choices. J Vasc Surg 2011;54(4): 1193–200.

40. Madan AK, Frantzides CT, Quiros R, et al. Effects of a laparoscopic course on student interest in surgical residency. JSLS 2005;9(2):134–7.

41. Wendel TM, Godellas CV, Prinz RA. Are there gender differences in choosing a surgical career? Surgery 2003;134(4):591–6 [discussion: 596–8].

42. Hill EJR, Bowman KA, Stalmeijer RE, et al. Can I cut it? Medical students' perceptions of surgeons and surgical careers. Am J Surg 2014;208(5):860–7.

43. Sanfey HA, Saalwachter-Schulman AR, Nyhof-Young JM, et al. Influences on medical student career choice: gender or generation? Arch Surg 2006;141(11):1086–94 [discussion: 1094].

44. Zarebczan B, Rajamanickam V, Lewis B, et al. The impact of the 80-hour work week on student interest in a surgical career. J Surg Res 2011;171(2):422–6.

45. Newton DA, Grayson MS, Thompson LF. The variable influence of lifestyle and income on medical students' career specialty choices: data from two U.S. medical schools, 1998-2004. Acad Med 2005;80(9):809–14.

46. Are C, Stoddard HA, O'Holleran B, et al. A multinational perspective on "lifestyle" and other perceptions of contemporary medical students about general surgery. Ann Surg 2012;256(2):378–86.

47. Zuccato JA, Kulkarni AV. The impact of early medical school surgical exposure on interest in neurosurgery. Can J Neurol Sci 2016;43(3):410–6.

48. Kaderli RM, Klasen JM, Businger AP. Mentoring in general surgery in Switzerland. Med Educ Online 2015;20:27528.

49. Montgomery SC, Privette AR, Ferguson PL, et al. Inadequately marketing our brand: medical student awareness of acute care surgery. J Trauma Acute Care Surg 2015;79(5):858–64.

50. Bell RM, Fann SA, Morrison JE, et al. Determining personal talents and behavioral styles of applicants to surgical training: a new look at an old problem, part II. J Surg Educ 2012;69(1):23–9.

51. Preece RA, Cope AC. Are surgeons born or made? A comparison of personality traits and learning styles between surgical trainees and medical students. J Surg Educ 2016;73(5):768–73.

52. Drosdeck JM, Osayi SN, Peterson LA, et al. Surgeon and nonsurgeon personalities at different career points. J Surg Res 2015;196(1):60–6.

53. Martinou E, Allan H, Vig S. Personality differences among junior postgraduate trainees in the United Kingdom. J Surg Educ 2015;72(1):122–7.

54. Eng MK, Macneily AE, Alden L. The urological personality: is it unique? Can J Urol 2004;11(5):2401–6.

55. McGreevy J, Wiebe D. A preliminary measurement of the surgical personality. Am J Surg 2002;184(2):121–5.

56. Thakur A, Fedorka P, Ko C, et al. Impact of mentor guidance in surgical career selection. J Pediatr Surg 2001;36(12):1802–4.

57. Sallee DS, Cooper C, Ravin CE. Medical student perceptions of diagnostic radiology. Influence of a senior radiology elective. Invest Radiol 1989;24(9):724–8.

58. Skrzypek M, Turska D. [Personality of medical students declaring surgical specialty choice in the context of prospective medical practice style]. Przegl Lek 2015;72(6):295–301.

59. Kiker BF, Zeh M. Relative income expectations, expected malpractice premium costs, and other determinants of physician specialty choice. J Health Soc Behav 1998;39(2):152–67.

60. Azizzadeh A, McCollum CH, Miller CC 3rd, et al. Factors influencing career choice among medical students interested in surgery. Curr Surg 2003;60(2): 210–3.

61. Stienen MN, Scholtes F, Samuel R, et al. Different but similar: personality traits of surgeons and internists-results of a cross-sectional observational study. BMJ Open 2018;8(7):e021310.

62. Hughes BD, Perone JA, Cummins CB, et al. Personality testing may identify applicants who will become successful in general surgery residency. J Surg Res 2019;233:240–8.

63. Schmidt LE, Cooper CA, Guo WA. Factors influencing US medical students' decision to pursue surgery. J Surg Res 2016;203(1):64–74.

64. Kozar RA, Anderson KD, Escobar-Chaves SL, et al. Preclinical students: who are surgeons? J Surg Res 2004;119(2):113–6.

65. Association of Women Surgeons. Association of Women Surgeons statement on gender salary equity. AOWS 2017. Available at: www.womensurgeons.org/2017-statement-on-gender-salaryequity/. Accessed May 1, 2017.

66. Richardson HC, Redfern N. Why do women reject surgical careers? Ann R Coll Surg Engl 2000;82(9 Suppl):290–3.

67. Gargiulo DA, Hyman NH, Hebert JC. Women in surgery: do we really understand the deterrents? Arch Surg 2006;141(4):405–7 [discussion: 407–8].

68. Park J, Minor S, Taylor RA, et al. Why are women deterred from general surgery training? Am J Surg 2005;190(1):141–6.

69. Lillemoe KD, Ahrendt GM, Yeo CJ, et al. Surgery–still an "old boys' club"? Surgery 1994;116(2):255–9 [discussion: 259–61].

70. Fitzgerald JE, Tang SW, Ravindra P, et al. Gender-related perceptions of careers in surgery among new medical graduates: results of a cross-sectional study. Am J Surg 2013;206(1):112–9.

71. Stratton TD, McLaughlin MA, Witte FM, et al. Does students' exposure to gender discrimination and sexual harassment in medical school affect specialty choice and residency program selection? Acad Med 2005;80(4):400–8.

72. Cochran A, Hauschild T, Elder WB, et al. Perceived gender-based barriers to careers in academic surgery. Am J Surg 2013;206(2):263–8.

73. Ku MC, Li YE, Prober C, et al. Decisions, decisions: how program diversity influences residency program choice. J Am Coll Surg 2011;213(2):294–305.

74. Dresler CM, Padgett DL, MacKinnon SE, et al. Experiences of women in cardiothoracic surgery. A gender comparison. Arch Surg 1996;131(11):1128–34 [discussion: 1135].

75. Schroen AT, Brownstein MR, Sheldon GF. Women in academic general surgery. Acad Med 2004;79(4):310–8.

76. Schroeder JE, Zisk-Rony RY, Liebergall M, et al. Medical students' and interns' interest in orthopedic surgery: the gender factor. J Surg Educ 2014;71(2): 198–204.

77. Calkins EV, Willoughby TL, Arnold LM. Women medical students' ratings of the required surgery clerkship: implications for career choice. J Am Med Womens Assoc 1992;47(2):58–60.

78. Hill E, Vaughan S. The only girl in the room: how paradigmatic trajectories deter female students from surgical careers. Med Educ 2013;47(6):547–56.

79. Ferris LE, Mackinnon SE, Mizgala CL, et al. Do Canadian female surgeons feel discriminated against as women? CMAJ 1996;154(1):21–7.

80. Jagsi R, Griffith KA, DeCastro RA, et al. Sex, role models, and specialty choices among graduates of US medical schools in 2006-2008. J Am Coll Surg 2014; 218(3):345–52.

81. Rouprêt M, Maggiori L, Lefevre JH. Upcoming female preponderance within surgery residents and the association of sex with the surgical career choice in the new millennium: results from a national survey in France. Am J Surg 2011; 202(2):237–42.

82. Snyder RA, Bills JL, Phillips SE, et al. Specific interventions to increase women's interest in surgery. J Am Coll Surg 2008;207(6):942–7, 947.e941-948.

# Evidence-Based Selection of Surgical Residents

Laurel A. Vaughan, MD, Jacob A. Quick, MD*

## KEYWORDS

- Recruitment • Resident • Selection • ABSITE • USMLE

## KEY POINTS

- It is crucial for programs to determine their unique desired applicant characteristics.
- Cognitive measures, such as letters of recommendation and United States Medical Licensing Examination step 2, may predict both academic and clinical success in residency.
- Noncognitive attributes, such as personality, grit, and personal interaction, may be the strongest predictors of overall residency success.
- Personal interviews, whether traditional or virtual, are crucial to establishing the concept of fit within a program.

## INTRODUCTION

The goal of every surgery residency selection committee should be to find candidates who have characteristics to become competent and safe surgeons. To identify ideal candidates, both cognitive achievements and noncognitive attributes must be examined. Programs may seek specific traits, but some qualities of accomplished surgeons are nearly universal:

- In-depth knowledge of medical pathophysiology and surgical techniques
- Benevolent and professional personality
- Strong communication skills
- Ability to work in teams
- Commitment to professional development
- Technical proficiency

Other characteristics are unique to individual programs. For example, one training program may seek out candidates with extensive research experience, whereas another may favor applicants with ties to the local community. It is imperative that

Department of Surgery, Division of Acute Care Surgery, University of Missouri, 1 Hospital Drive, MC220, Columbia, MO 65212, USA
* Corresponding author.
E-mail address: quickja@health.missouri.edu
Twitter: @LaurelAVaughan (L.A.V.); @jakequickmd (J.A.Q.)

Surg Clin N Am 101 (2021) 667–677
https://doi.org/10.1016/j.suc.2021.05.012
0039-6109/21/© 2021 Elsevier Inc. All rights reserved.

surgical.theclinics.com

programs first decide on these desired characteristics, and develop a recruitment plan to fulfill them.

There are 2 main components of the residency applicant's dossier: application and interview. Pinpointing match-worthy candidates from an increasingly deep and similar applicant pool can be daunting, and begins with application review. Cognitive achievements appearing in the Electronic Residency Application Service(ERAS) application are often easily stratified and make up most of the paper application. These cognitive achievements include United States Medical Licensing Examination (USMLE) scores, clerkship academic performance reviews, Medical Student Performance Evaluation, letters of recommendations, medical school grades, personal statement, publications/presentations, and extracurricular activities. These metrics predominantly assess knowledge and academic aptitudes, and form the basis for interview selection. The 2020 National Residency Matching Program (NRMP) Program Directors survey examined factors that program directors use to select applicants for an interview. The 4 most common factors cited in selecting applicants to interview are [1,2]:

- USMLE step 1 score
- Letters of recommendation in the specialty
- USMLE step 2 Clinical Knowledge (CK) score
- Personal statement

However, when ranking applicants, the 4 most common factors cited from the NRMP Program Directors survey are largely noncognitive[1]:

- Interpersonal skills
- Interactions with faculty during interview
- Interactions with house staff during interview
- Feedback from current residents

This list suggests that noncognitive factors strongly influence ranking candidates.[3] It also highlights the perceived importance of both applicant components. Cognitive successes are frequently used to determine an applicant's ability to succeed academically, whereas the interview is used to determine fit within a specific program. In layman's terms, many use the paper application to answer the question, "Can the candidate make it?" However, the interview answers, "Can the candidate make it here?" This article examines evidence-based recruitment factors consistent with excelling in surgical training.

## DISCUSSION
### Candidate Selection: Cognitive Achievements and the Application

**USMLE step 1 and step 2 clinical knowledge scores predict academic performance in residency**

Program directors commonly cite the USMLE step 1 score as the most important factor in selecting applicants for an interview.[1] Several studies have shown a relationship between higher USMLE scores and American Board of Surgery (ABS) In-training Examination (ABSITE), as well as first-time ABS Qualifying Examination pass rates.[2,4–6] Studies evaluating the relationship of USMLE scores with clinical performance during residency have been mixed.[6–8] Several studies suggest the lack of correlation between USMLE step 1 and clinical success is because the examination is not designed to test clinical skill acquisition.[8] However, other studies have shown that USMLE step 1 scores do correlate with improved manual dexterity, suggesting some academic crossover to the noncognitive realm of success.[6,9]

USMLE step 1 becomes a pass/fail test in January 2022, potentially creating additional challenges. The scoring change was proposed to encourage a more balanced assessment of interviewees.[10] Several studies have evaluated program director perspectives regarding the change to pass/fail, and found that most program directors disagreed with the scoring change and thought that it will make it more difficult to objectively compare applicants. Program directors also stated that this change will shift the emphasis to USMLE step 2 CK score.[11–13]

Despite several studies showing surgical program director disapproval of the USMLE's 2022 scoring changes, it may be a blessing in disguise. Like USMLE step 1, step 2 CK scores do seem to be predictive of academic performance in residency.[5,8,14,15] Maker and colleagues[16] showed that residents with higher step 2 CK scores are more likely to pass the ABS Certifying Examination. Although step 2 CK scores lack overall correlation with leadership ability, they do correlate with both patient care and interpersonal and communication skills milestones, suggesting a stronger link to clinical performance than step 1.[17,18]

### Medical school performance/grades predict academic performance in residency
Much like USMLE score, medical school grades and clinical clerkship evaluations have shown correlation to ABS examination scores, but do not significantly predict clinical performance during residency.[2,6,7,19]

Grade inflation has become an increasingly widespread issue that can confound the validity of using preclerkship and clerkship grades as determinants for interview invitation.[20–23] Grading variability, both between schools and within schools, results in wide-ranging possibilities in which graders can delineate and document either poor or superior performance.[24] Further, assigning meaning to these scores/grades is an even more daunting task when evaluating applicants. Several methods to combat grade variability have been suggested, but they have yet to be universally implemented.[25]

### Letters of recommendation predict clinical performance
Multiple studies have examined what make a letter great. These factors include personal relationships with letter writers, certain key descriptors used (such as outstanding, or superior), and medical school of origin.[2] One of the most important concepts a letter can convey is the desire to train the applicant. The phrases "We plan to recruit this candidate," or "I give my highest recommendation" have been shown to be the most important phrases in letters.[26] Using the 6 core competencies, outlined by the Accreditation Council on Graduate Medical Education (ACGME), to define clinical performance success, several studies have shown letters of recommendation to be predictive of clinical performance.[2,18] Further, global performance metrics have also strongly correlated with letter quality, suggesting that letters of recommendation are a key component to determining future success.[27]

However, letters of recommendation are fallible. Applicants choose their letter writers, who may inflate applicant performance, creating challenges in deciphering the applicants' true abilities.[28] Standardized letters of recommendation have attempted to diminish these issues; however, many investigators argue that standardized letters actually worsen performance inflation.[29] Instead, some suggest that letters should include the context in which letter writers know the student, character and personality traits of the applicant, along with any red flags or professionalism issues and an overall recommendation.[30]

### Prior nonmedical success predicts future medical success
Participating in extracurricular activities, such as team sports, is clearly desired by many surgical program directors.[31] It is common for programs to seek individuals

who have excelled at something outside of medicine. Whether it be playing a musical instrument, participating in sports, or showing entrepreneurship, excelling at a high level in some other arena before medicine is an indicator of drive, will, determination, and grit. In a study of general surgery residents, those who had a unique skill were more likely not only to complete a surgical residency but also to perform well.[7] Similarly, a history of playing team sports has inversely correlated with attrition, and predicted success.[32,33] It is not only the presence of a specific preexisting skill set but the effort that it took to reach proficiency of that skill that is important. Of equal importance is possessing the passion for a surgical career, just as the candidate may have shown passion for a prior achievement. This point is where the cognitive and noncognitive domains cross over to begin to form an overall impression of a surgical residency applicant.

## Candidate Selection: Noncognitive Abilities and the Interview

### Manual dexterity is more than hand-eye coordination
Surgical selection has not conventionally included dexterity evaluation, even though this attribute is important to surgical practice.[34] Some programs have begun including dexterity and psychomotor assessments in the selection process to improve engagement and robustness of the process.[35,36] Although some studies show correlations between dexterity and clinical performance only in novices, others have shown a high degree of correlation with operative skill at the end of training.[37,38] Further, applicants with a high baseline level of dexterity progress quicker in training, and therefore graduate as more competent surgeons.[39,40] In contrast, those who lack manual psychomotor skills may consume more educational resources, take longer to meet educational goals, and may divert education from other trainees. These studies suggest that dexterity and surgical skill testing should be included in the interview process.

### Personality testing predicts success
Personality assessments may be beneficial in determining future success and identifying red flags in applications. For example, the narcissism personality index may be used to identify maladaptive behaviors before meeting candidates in the interview.[41] The Myers-Briggs "intuitive" and "think" preferences have been shown to be associated with later success in a surgical career.[2] Emotional intelligence, defined as a disposition or ability of individuals to perceive and process the emotions of themselves and others, has been linked to favorable outcomes in the business world and also more recently in the health care arena. The Trait Emotional Intelligence Questionnaire (TEIQue) has shown correlations between emotional intelligence and final rank position, and suggests emotional intelligence is a desired characteristic.[42] Higher emotional intelligence scores have also been correlated to improved performance, enhanced well-being, and less burnout in residency training.[42–44]

The Big 5 personality traits have been used to predict successful residents through identification of extroversion, conscientiousness, and emotional stability.[45] The Big 5 are frequently combined with grit analyses. Individuals with high levels of grit have high tendencies to persevere through short-term setbacks, and are focused to achieve their future goals. The Big 5 and the Grit Scale have been studied in many industries during the recruitment phase of employment, with both showing correlations to later success.[45–48] Grit also seems to delineate desirable personality characteristics. A recent meta-analysis of grit studies found that, although grit by itself was not strongly correlated with performance, it was very strongly correlated with conscientiousness, a characteristic found in successful surgeons.[49] Following Duckworth and colleague's[46] publication on grit, testing for grit and other personality traits has significantly increased. This increase has sparked concerns over applicants purposefully skewing answers toward perceived desirable answers. This phenomenon is not new and has been extensively studied in the business and psychology literature.[50,51] Most experts agree that, in general, individuals skew their scores to portray themselves in a positive manner. Despite the human tendency to please, personality tests still remain a valid quantitative measure to delineate desirable personality characteristics of applicants for surgical residency.

### Preinterview materials focus recruitment efforts

Preinterview questionnaires and assessments have been used in business for many years. Preinterview assessments may reduce the number of interviewees and improve the ability to match those interviewed. In this way, preinterview questionnaires can allow a more focused approach. Recently, the potential benefits of preinterview assessments, whether they be questionnaires, essays, knowledge or personality examinations, or institution-specific supplemental applications, have been realized by residency programs. Completion rates are typically high, and individuals who do not complete the assessments typically have lower standardized test scores, and are likely less-desired candidates.[52] Therefore, preinterview material completion may self-select candidates with a higher likelihood of matching at any individual program.

### The interview

Much has been written about the concept of fit, when discussing job performance and placement. Remarkably accurate assessments can be made in a short period of time when determining whether a candidate is right for a program. The difficulty lies within the definition of what fit and right mean from a quantitative standpoint. Although numerical scoring is nearly impossible when describing an intangible feeling, there are data to support the gut instincts of interviewers. Thin slicing is a concept of taking small segments or fragments of information and making immediate over-arching decisions.[53] Surgeons are typically accustomed to thin slicing, because they do it frequently during emergency procedures or situations, where rapid decisions are made based on limited information. Multiple studies in a variety of disciplines have shown a high degree of predictable candidate success, or failure, after a brief interaction.[54–57] Some have shown that accurate predictions can be made even after viewing a single still photograph of a candidate.[54] These findings emphasize the importance of personal interaction during the residency recruitment process, and highlights the necessity of interviews.

Despite the impressive accuracy of the interviewer's initial reaction to a candidate, traditional face-to-face interviews have inherent issues with subjectivity, reliability, and interviewer concordance. Multiple attempts have been made to normalize these issues, including using group interview techniques, structured interviews, behavioral questioning ,and blinded interviews.[58–60] Group interviews can save time and money, and have become increasingly common, because they allow programs to assess the interaction within the group of candidates and with the interviewer. Clinical (behavioral) scenarios are often used, and teamwork, as well as communication and problem-solving skills, can be assessed.[61] Structured interviews can decrease the variability of interview reactions and improve concordance by assigning questions or topics to individual interviewers.[62] The behavioral interview method seems readily amenable to assess for emotional intelligence.[59] Behavioral interviews typically provide a clinical scenario, often with no correct answer, and ask candidates to describe their approaches to the problem. Questions can be customized to target emotional intelligence facets that are considered essential in a surgical trainee. Blinding interviewers to application data, such as USMLE scores, effectively decreases biases toward cognitive measures, such as grades and scores.[63–65] Although bias favoring academic success is limited by blinding, it can be argued that it should not be. After all, a key component to overall success is academic success.[66]

### Virtual interviews

With the recent pandemic, virtual interviews and interactions have become widespread, which presents multiple issues with resident recruitment. First, the virtual environment can be cumbersome for programs and candidates alike. Second, technical aspects of conducting mass virtual interviews are typically outside the realm of expertise for many program directors and coordinators. Third, traditional interviews are costly to the candidates, and thus were self-limited in number by financial constraints. With virtual interviews, there is very little cost or time added for each subsequent virtual interview.[67] This serious consequence will undoubtedly lead to programs being flooded with candidate applications, and will create difficulties in deciding who to interview, who has a real interest in the program, and who to rank.[68]

Virtual preapplication meetings using social media platforms have been a way for programs to determine the interest of applicants. The generally informal virtual meet-and-greets typically address some frequently asked questions and allow candidates to learn more about an individual program before applying,[69] which bodes well for both parties. Limited experience has shown some positive results, and typically are best when the groups are small.[70] Virtual happy hours, as they are sometimes referred to, may also help fill the void left by the lack of the preinterview dinner.

Panel interviews have also made a comeback in the virtual environment, likely because of the ease of structure. A panel interview may consist of multiple, or even all, faculty members interviewing a single candidate. From a candidate standpoint, this can increase anxiety. From a program standpoint, it allows a single interview to be conducted for each candidate, which may streamline the rank process, which is often completed immediately following interviews. Single interviews may be added to diversify the interview day.[71]

## SUMMARY

Every year surgery residency programs are tasked with recruiting ideal residency applicants. The task of teasing out those individuals who will excel in surgery is challenging, because most medical students are already high performers. This article suggests that many criteria used during recruitment have both benefits and detriments to the process. One likely explanation is the vast differences in focus between residency programs. What makes a great resident in one program may not do so in another program. Once a program determines what is important, then the task of identifying those characteristics begins.

Using components of the application and interview, commonly sought-after attributes, such as academic prowess, technical and communication skills, professionalism, and benevolence, may be identified. USMLE step 2 CK scores are useful to determine both current and future academic performance, as well as clinical performance.[6–8,18] Strong letters of recommendation and excellence in extracurricular activities before medical school should also be emphasized during application review because they both showed positive correlation to future resident performance.

Once the cognitive abilities of an applicant meet a program's standards, the personal interview is an effective way to delve into the applicants personality and identify any red flags that may hinder the applicant's achievement during residency.[41]

Extroversion, conscientiousness, emotional stability, and high emotional intelligence scores have been correlated to improved performance, enhanced well-being, and less burnout in residency training.[42–45]

The interview remains essential, because a remarkably accurate assessment of fit can be made in a short period of time. To help determine whether a candidate is the right fit, programs can use group, blinded, behavioral, or structured interviews.[59,61,62] With the recent pandemic, virtual interviews are becoming common, and retain both the good and bad traits of traditional interviews.

## DISCLOSURE

The authors have nothing to disclose.

## REFERENCES

1. National Resident Matching Program. Results of the 2020 NRMP Program Director Survey [Internet]. Available at: https://mk0nrmp3oyqui6wqfm.kinstacdn.com/wp-content/uploads/2020/08/2020-PD-Survey.pdf. Accessed September 22, 2020.

2. Brothers TE, Wetherholt S. Importance of the faculty interview during the resident application process. J Surg Educ 2007;64(6):378–85.

3. Shebrain S, Arafeh M, Munene G, et al. The role of academic achievements and psychometric measures in the ranking process. Am J Surg 2019;217(3):568–71.

4. Sutton E, Richardson JD, Ziegler C, et al. Is USMLE Step 1 score a valid predictor of success in surgical residency? Am J Surg 2014;208(6):1029–34 [discussion: 1034].

5. de Virgilio C, Yaghoubian A, Kaji A, et al. Predicting performance on the American Board of Surgery qualifying and certifying examinations: a multi-institutional study. Arch Surg 2010;145(9):852–6.

6. Bell JG, Kanellitsas I, Shaffer L. Selection of obstetrics and gynecology residents on the basis of medical school performance. Am J Obstet Gynecol 2002;186(5):1091–4.

7. Alterman DM, Jones TM, Heidel RE, et al. The predictive value of general surgery application data for future resident performance. J Surg Educ 2011;68(6):513–8.

8. McGaghie WC, Cohen ER, Wayne DB. Are United States Medical Licensing Exam Step 1 and 2 scores valid measures for postgraduate medical residency selection decisions? Acad Med J Assoc Am Med Coll 2011;86(1):48–52.

9. Goldberg AE, Neifeld JP, Wolfe LG, et al. Correlation of manual dexterity with USMLE scores and medical student class rank. J Surg Res 2008;147(2):212–5.

10. United States Medical Licensing Examination. Summary report and preliminary recommendations from the invitational conference on USMLE Scoring(InCUS). 2019.

11. Pontell ME, Makhoul AT, Ganesh Kumar N, et al. The Change of USMLE Step 1 to Pass/Fail: Perspectives of the Surgery Program Director. J Surg Educ 2020;78(1):91–8.

12. Cohn MR, Bigach SD, Bernstein DN, et al. Resident selection in the wake of united states medical licensing examination step 1 transition to pass/fail scoring. J Am Acad Orthop Surg 2020;28(21):865–73.

13. Chisholm LP, Drolet BC. USMLE step 1 scoring changes and the urology residency application process: program directors' perspectives. Urology 2020;145:79–82.

14. Rayamajhi S, Dhakal P, Wang L, et al. Do USMLE steps, and ITE score predict the American Board of Internal Medicine Certifying Exam results? BMC Med Educ 2020;20(1):79.

15. Shellito JL, Osland JS, Helmer SD, et al. American Board of Surgery examinations: can we identify surgery residency applicants and residents who will pass the examinations on the first attempt? Am J Surg 2010;199(2):216–22.

16. Maker VK, Zahedi MM, Villines D, et al. Can we predict which residents are going to pass/fail the oral boards? J Surg Educ 2012;69(6):705–13.

17. Cohen ER, Goldstein JL, Schroedl CJ, et al. Are USMLE Scores Valid Measures for Chief Resident Selection? J Grad Med Educ 2020;12(4):441–6.

18. Hayek SA, Wickizer AP, Lane SM, et al. Application Factors May Not Be Predictors of Success Among General Surgery Residents as Measured by ACGME Milestones. J Surg Res 2020;253:34–40.

19. Raman T, Alrabaa RG, Sood A, et al. Does Residency Selection Criteria Predict Performance in Orthopaedic Surgery Residency? Clin Orthop 2016;474(4):908–14.

20. Fazio SB, Papp KK, Torre DM, et al. Grade inflation in the internal medicine clerkship: a national survey. Teach Learn Med 2013;25(1):71–6.

21. Cacamese SM, Elnicki M, Speer AJ. Grade inflation and the internal medicine subinternship: a national survey of clerkship directors. Teach Learn Med 2007;19(4):343–6.

22. Alexander EK, Osman NY, Walling JL, et al. Variation and imprecision of clerkship grading in U.S. medical schools. Acad Med J Assoc Am Med Coll 2012;87(8):1070–6.

23. Bowen RES, Grant WJ, Schenarts KD. The sum is greater than its parts: clinical evaluations and grade inflation in the surgery clerkship. Am J Surg 2015;209(4):760–4.

24. Takayama H, Grinsell R, Brock D, et al. Is it appropriate to use core clerkship grades in the selection of residents? Curr Surg 2006;63(6):391–6.

25. Lipman JM, Schenarts KD. Defining Honors in the Surgery Clerkship. J Am Coll Surg 2016;223(4):665–9.

26. Rajesh A, Rivera M, Asaad M, et al. What Are We REALLY Looking for in a Letter of Recommendation? J Surg Educ 2019;76(6):e118–24.

27. Bhat R, Takenaka K, Levine B, et al. Predictors of a Top Performer During Emergency Medicine Residency. J Emerg Med 2015;49(4):505–12.

28. Hegarty CB, Lane DR, Love JN, et al. Council of emergency medicine residency directors standardized letter of recommendation writers' questionnaire. J Grad Med Educ 2014;6(2):301–6.

29. Jackson JS, Bond M, Love JN, et al. Emergency Medicine Standardized Letter of Evaluation (SLOE): Findings From the New Electronic SLOE Format. J Grad Med Educ 2019;11(2):182–6.

30. Naples R, French JC, Lipman JM. Best practices in letters of recommendation for general surgery residency: results of expert stakeholder focus groups. J Surg Educ 2020;77(6):e121–31.

31. Chole RA, Ogden MA. Predictors of future success in otolaryngology residency applicants. Arch Otolaryngol Head Neck Surg 2012;138(8):707–12.

32. Kohanzadeh S, Hayase Y, Lefor MK, et al. Factors affecting attrition in graduate surgical education. Am Surg 2007;73(10):963–6.

33. Egol KA, Collins J, Zuckerman JD. Success in orthopaedic training: resident selection and predictors of quality performance. J Am Acad Orthop Surg 2011;19(2):72–80.

34. Gallagher AG, Leonard G, Traynor OJ. Role and feasibility of psychomotor and dexterity testing in selection for surgical training. ANZ J Surg 2009;79(3): 108–13.

35. Gallagher AG, Neary P, Gillen P, et al. Novel method for assessment and selection of trainees for higher surgical training in general surgery. ANZ J Surg 2008;78(4): 282–90.

36. Carroll SM, Kennedy AM, Traynor O, et al. Objective assessment of surgical performance and its impact on a national selection programme of candidates for higher surgical training in plastic surgery. J Plast Reconstr Aesthet Surg 2009; 62(12):1543–9.

37. Wanzel KR, Hamstra SJ, Caminiti MF, et al. Visual-spatial ability correlates with efficiency of hand motion and successful surgical performance. Surgery 2003; 134(5):750–7.

38. Maan ZN, Maan IN, Darzi AW, et al. Systematic review of predictors of surgical performance. Br J Surg 2012;99(12):1610–21.

39. Jardine D, Hoagland B, Perez A, et al. Evaluation of Surgical Dexterity During the Interview Day: Another Factor for Consideration. J Grad Med Educ 2015;7(2): 234–7.

40. Buckley CE, Kavanagh DO, Nugent E, et al. The impact of aptitude on the learning curve for laparoscopic suturing. Am J Surg 2014;207(2):263–70.

41. Gawad N, Ibrahim AM, Duffy M, et al. Going beyond the numerical scoresheet: identifying maladaptive narcissistic traits in residency applicants. J Surg Educ 2019;76(1):65–76.

42. Lin DT, Kannappan A, Lau JN. The assessment of emotional intelligence among candidates interviewing for general surgery residency. J Surg Educ 2013;70(4): 514–21.

43. Talarico JF, Varon AJ, Banks SE, et al. Emotional intelligence and the relationship to resident performance: a multi-institutional study. J Clin Anesth 2013;25(3): 181–7.

44. Gleason F, Baker SJ, Wood T, et al. Emotional Intelligence and Burnout in Surgical Residents: A 5-Year Study. J Surg Educ 2020;77(6):e63–70.

45. Hughes BD, Perone JA, Cummins CB, et al. Personality Testing May Identify Applicants Who Will Become Successful in General Surgery Residency. J Surg Res 2019;233:240–8.

46. Duckworth AL, Peterson C, Matthews MD, et al. Grit: perseverance and passion for long-term goals. J Pers Soc Psychol 2007;92(6):1087–101.

47. Eskreis-Winkler L, Shulman EP, Beal SA, et al. The grit effect: predicting retention in the military, the workplace, school and marriage. Front Psychol 2014;5:36.

48. Burkhart RA, Tholey RM, Guinto D, et al. Grit: a marker of residents at risk for attrition? Surgery 2014;155(6):1014–22.

49. Credé M, Tynan MC, Harms PD. Much ado about grit: A meta-analytic synthesis of the grit literature. J Pers Soc Psychol 2017;113(3):492–511.

50. Melchers KG, Roulin N, Buehl A. A review of applicant faking in selection interviews. Int J Sel Assess 2020;28(2):123–42.

51. Birkeland SA, Manson TM, Kisamore JL, et al. A meta-analytic investigation of job applicant faking on personality measures: job applicant faking on personality measures. Int J Sel Assess 2006;14(4):317–35.

52. Gardner AK, Cavanaugh KJ, Willis RE, et al. If You Build It, Will They Come? Candidate Completion of Preinterview Screening Assessments. J Surg Educ 2019;76(6):1534–8.

53. Gladwell M. Blink: the power of thinking without thinking. New York: Little, Brown and Co.; 2005.

54. Schmidt G. The effect of thin slicing on structured interview decisions. Grad Theses Diss [Internet]. 2007. Available at: https://scholarcommons.usf.edu/etd/2356. Accessed October 8, 2020.

55. Murphy NA, Hall JA, Ruben MA, et al. Predictive Validity of Thin-Slice Nonverbal Behavior from Social Interactions. Pers Soc Psychol Bull 2019;45(7):983–93.

56. Nguyen LS, Gatica-Perez D. I Would Hire You in a Minute: Thin Slices of Nonverbal Behavior in Job Interviews. In: Proceedings of the 2015 ACM on International Conference on Multimodal Interaction - ICMI '15 [Internet]. Seattle, Washington, USA: ACM Press; 2015 [cited 2020 Oct 8]. p. 51–8. Available at: http://dl.acm.org/citation.cfm?doid=2818346.2820760. Accessed October 8, 2020.

57. Ambady N, Bernieri FJ, Richeson JA. Toward a histology of social behavior: judgmental accuracy from thin slices of the behavioral stream. In: Advances in Experimental social psychology. Cambridge (MA): Academic Press Elsevier; 2000. p. 201–71. Available at: https://linkinghub.elsevier.com/retrieve/pii/S0065260100800064. Accessed October 8, 2020.

58. Lin DT, Liebert CA, Tran J, et al. Emotional Intelligence as a Predictor of Resident Well-Being. J Am Coll Surg 2016;223(2):352–8.

59. Easdown LJ, Castro PL, Shinkle EP, et al. The behavioral interview, a method to evaluate acgme competencies in resident selection: a pilot project. J Educ Perioper Med 2005;7(1):E032.

60. Kiraly L, Dewey E, Brasel K. Hawks and doves: adjusting for bias in residency interview scoring. J Surg Educ 2020;77(6):e132–7.

61. Smooke D. Group Interviewing: Efficient Solution or Ineffective Evaluation? [Internet]. MightyRecruiter. 2017. Available at: https://www.mightyrecruiter.com/blog/group-interviewing-efficient-solution-or-ineffective-evaluation/. Accessed October 8, 2020.

62. Association of American Medical Colleges. Best Practices for Conducting Residency Program Interviews [Internet]. 2016. Available at: https://www.aamc.org/system/files/2020-05/best%20practices%20for%20conducting%20residency%20program%20interviews.pdf. Accessed October 8, 2020.

63. Swanson WS, Harris MC, Master C, et al. The impact of the interview in pediatric residency selection. Ambul Pediatr 2005;5(4):216–20.

64. Brustman LE, Williams FL, Carroll K, et al. The effect of blinded versus nonblinded interviews in the resident selection process. J Grad Med Educ 2010;2(3):349–53.

65. Stephenson-Famy A, Houmard BS, Oberoi S, et al. Use of the Interview in Resident Candidate Selection: A Review of the Literature. J Grad Med Educ 2015; 7(4):539–48.

66. Hauge LS, Stroessner SJ, Chowdhry S, et al, Association for Surgical Education. Evaluating resident candidates: does closed file review impact faculty ratings? Am J Surg 2007;193(6):761–5.

67. Bamba R, Bhagat N, Tran PC, et al. Virtual interviews for the independent plastic surgery match: a modern convenience or a modern misrepresentation? J Surg Educ 2020;78(2):612–21.

68. Patel TY, Bedi HS, Deitte LA, et al. Brave New World: Challenges and Opportunities in the COVID-19 Virtual Interview Season. Acad Radiol 2020;27(10):1456–60.

69. Rajesh A, Asaad M. Alternative Strategies for Evaluating General Surgery Residency Applicants and an Interview Limit for MATCH 2021: An Impending Necessity. Ann Surg 2020;273(1):109–11.

70. Hill MV, Bleicher RJ, Farma JM. A how-to guide: virtual interviews in the era of social distancing. J Surg Educ 2020;78(1):321–3.

71. Vining CC, Eng OS, Hogg ME, et al. Virtual Surgical Fellowship Recruitment During COVID-19 and Its Implications for Resident/Fellow Recruitment in the Future. Ann Surg Oncol 2020;27(Suppl 3):911–5.

# Value of Standardized Testing in Surgical Training

Amy Han, MD, Judith French, PhD, Jeremy Lipman, MD, MHPE*

## KEYWORDS

- Surgical education • Resident assessment • Standardized testing • Certification

## KEY POINTS

- Standardized testing undergoes rigorous psychometric analysis to ensure validity and reality of the examination.
- Standardized tests add value to assessment of surgical trainees by offering objective comparison among trainees on a national level.
- Limitations of standardized testing includes poor test-takers, biases, and financial burden.

## BACKGROUND

Assessment is a cornerstone of surgical education. As producers of the next generation of general surgeons, surgical educators have created a system of assessment to illustrate to stakeholders that our graduates are deserving of the title "surgeon." A major component of that assessment system is standardized testing. For decades testing standardization has served as a key method for identifying surgical competence.[1] Even before entering surgical education, trainees are well versed in the intricacies of standardized testing whether through primary or secondary school, college entrance examinations, or even the Medical College Admission Test. In this section the authors take a closer look at standardized testing in surgical education to provide an overview of its many influences in determining who will earn the title "surgeon." First, they begin by describing what is encompassed by the phrase standardized test.

## DEFINING STANDARDIZED TESTING

Standardized testing indicates an examination is administered, scored, and interpreted in the same manner for all participants, regardless of the testing location.[2] The tests can be composed of multiple choice questions (MCQs), short answer, true/false, or even demonstrations of clinical skills. The examination results can be norm referenced or criterion referenced. Norm-referenced result indicates one's test

Cleveland Clinic, Department of General Surgery, 9500 Euclid Avenue, Cleveland, OH 44195, USA
* Corresponding author.
E-mail address: lipmanj@ccf.org

Surg Clin N Am 101 (2021) 679–691
https://doi.org/10.1016/j.suc.2021.05.013
0039-6109/21/© 2021 Elsevier Inc. All rights reserved.

surgical.theclinics.com

results are compared with other test takers, whereas criterion-referenced results show a test taker has met established performance metrics irrespective of other examinees.[3] Regardless of the interpretation type of the results the ultimate goal of a standardized test is to serve as a "stamp of approval" an individual meets set requirements. In order to achieve this level of acceptability and trust these tests undergo various methods to establish evidence for validity and reliability.

High-stakes standardized tests, which place a great burden on failure, must undergo rigorous research to support validity evidence and show the results are repeatable (reliable).[4] These tests tend to be developed by testing experts and are resource intensive to create. Lower stakes tests, which have fewer consequences for poor performance, must still undergo research to support validity and reliability, but the depth of evidence is often not at the same level as high-stakes examinations.[3] Whether high- or low-stakes standardized tests, developers need the examination to be true to its purpose and to measure what is intended. A classic example of a standardized test straying from its purpose is a mathematics test designed to measure ability to multiply double digit numbers, but because the questions are presented as word problems the examination becomes a test of reading ability instead.

## CREATING A STANDARDIZED EXAMINATION

So how does one go about creating a standardized test that sticks to its original intent and possesses evidence for validity and reliability? There is no "one-size-fits-all" method; however, there are general guidelines aspiring designers can follow. Test creators must start out determining the goal or purpose of the test to ensure the overall scope of what will be included and what will be excluded.[5] Once the goal is defined, the type of standardized test can be selected so that the test structure aligns with the test purpose. For example, if the purpose of the examination is to test communication skills in a trainee, a multiple choice test may not be the best fit. However, MCQs could pair well with an examination focused on ascertaining trainees' medical knowledge of treatment of small bowel obstruction. The type of standardized test selected will then determine the next step of creating items to be used on the examination. Short answer response, MCQs, and even manual skills criteria need to be created to assess all concepts determined by the original scope of the test. These items must undergo rigorous scrutiny from content experts, statisticians, and sample test populations. For many standardized tests item response theory (IRT), a psychometric model that links learner performance to item difficulty, provides the framework for this scrutiny.[6] Finally, as standardized tests are used they require continued monitoring and altering to ensure the examinations remain true to their purpose and do not develop unforeseen issues.

## HISTORICAL CONTEXT FOR STANDARDIZED TESTING IN SURGICAL TRAINING

Surgical training evolved significantly from the days of an apprenticeship model where graduated responsibility was granted as summarized by "see one, do one, teach one" famously indoctrinated by William Halsted. Today, training programs are established and maintained with standards set by Accreditation Council of Graduate Medical Education (ACGME) that balances patient safety and trainee well-being and reduces health care costs.[7] Founded in 1937, the American Board of Surgery (ABS) is an independent, nonprofit organization that established a certification process to safeguard the public through its board certification process for surgeons to recognize those who demonstrate "commitment to professionalism, lifelong learning, and quality patient care."[8] ABS sets the standards for granting certification to candidates seeking initial or maintenance of certification in surgery.[9] ABS carries out this function through assessments of fundamental knowledge essential for the diagnosis and treatment of surgical conditions, clinical judgment, and decision-making.[9] ABS also diligently works to maintain the public perception and faith that the examinations are valid and reliable with high integrity to maintain high standards of quality surgical care.[9] ABS's Assessment Committee actively monitors its examinations for any suspicious or irregular behaviors such as better performance on previously used questions that may suggest the integrity of the examination is compromised.

## PURPOSE OF STANDARDIZED TESTING IN SURGICAL TRAINING

As highlighted by Epstein,[8] the goals of assessment in medical education can be divided into 3 broad categories:

1. Providing learners and instructors the motivation and guidance for future learning
2. Public safety
3. Promotion to the next training level—promotion through residency training, board certification, and continuing medical education for certification maintenance.

The purpose of standardized testing in surgical training measures the individual trainees' medical knowledge, technical skills, and competency to graduate from training as well as the effectiveness of the training program's educational curriculum and how each program compares with other training programs.[9,10] Standardized testing has long held an important position in surgical training; this extends from the National Board of Medical Examiners (NBME) subject examination in surgery through maintenance of certification examinations used by ABS. The original intended use for many of these tests has been supplemented or supplanted to meet the evolving needs of educators and administrators. These changes have led to a variety of sequelae.

## DESCRIPTIONS OF EXAMPLES OF STANDARDIZED TESTING IN SURGICAL EDUCATION
### National Board of Medical Examiners Surgery Subject Tests

The NBME subject examination in surgery is usually the first standardized examination specific to surgical education encountered by a learner. Typically, this test is administered at the conclusion of the core clerkship in surgery and is intended to be a high-quality, efficient, cost-effective assessment to promote improved learning and instruction.[11] The examination consists of 110 MCQs that assess the examinee's foundation of medical knowledge and diagnostic workup as well as management of surgical disease processes. Many institutions use the NBME surgery examination as a component of final clerkship grade determination, as it allows for comparison of an examinee's performance to the national normative data.[12] A correlation has been observed between the NBME surgery examination score in surgery and eventual matriculation to a residency program in a surgical specialty.[13] This observation may be related to students who attain high grades on their surgical clerkship being more competitive for those specialties. Alternatively, though, it may be that after achieving a lower grade on the clerkship students are discouraged from applying into the field. The final clerkship grade is often formulated through amalgamation of many subjective assessments, with the NBME surgery examination as one of the few objective determinants. Poor correlation has been observed, however, between the NBME surgery examination and other measures of medical knowledge.[14]

In addition, the NBME surgery examination is a national, standardized test and thus does not take into account the wide variability of curricular content across core surgery clerkships at different institutions. The value of a standardized test to assess nonstandardized curricula is questionable. However, although the grading is normalized to other medical students nationally, there is not a defined passing score, and thus institutions are empowered to apply the test results as they find appropriate. The creation of a medical student core curriculum by the American College of Surgeons (ACS) and Association for Surgical Education now provides a framework on which to align both the instruction and assessment of medical student knowledge in a standardized manner.[15]

### American College of Surgeons—Entering Residency Readiness Assessment

The American College of Surgeons Entering Residency Readiness Assessment was created by the ACS Division of Education as an online, case-based formative instrument to measure entering resident's preparedness with emphasis on clinical decision-making skills for clinical scenarios commonly encountered by junior residents.[16] It has undergone psychometrically rigorous measures of key skills needed for entering residents to safely assume their new clinical responsibilities. Case-based scenarios assess clinical decision-making skills, not their ability to simply recall factual knowledge. This formative assessment is intended to be used to devise learning plans that address areas in need of reinforcement for individual residents or the entering group as a whole.[17] The score report includes a template to facilitate creating an individualized learning plan, supporting its role as a strictly formative tool. In addition, it has been suggested that decisions on the required level of supervision may be informed by these results.[17]

### Advanced Trauma Life Support

Advanced Trauma Life Support (ATLS) is a worldwide program that teaches a concise, standardized method to provide care for a trauma patient.[18] Graduating surgery residents are required by the ABS to have taken and passed the ATLS course but are not required to have current certification.[19] The program consists of 2 assessments: an initial assessment skills station and a written posttest. The initial assessment skills station is a hands-on examination where the test taker must perform an initial assessment on a trauma patient; this requires the examinee to reach certain predetermined "critical treatment decisions" and perform specific psychomotor skills (eg, intubation) on a simulated or standardized patient. There are 21 possible patient scenarios but the method with which they are assessed is the same using a yes or no checklist.[20] The written posttest is a 40 MCQ examination that assesses test taker's medical knowledge of ATLS concepts and must be passed with a minimum 75% score. ATLS participants are allowed to retake both assessments on the day of the course if needed.

Because of the graduation requirement and the potential employer requirement depending on the position, ATLS is considered a high-stakes examination. The MCQ portion has undergone psychometric testing to provide some validity evidence to support its high-stakes nature.[21,22] Although some potential bias of the program's assessments has been identified, to date the MCQs have not undergone differential item functioning (DIF) to further elucidate this finding.[23]

### Fundamentals of Laparoscopic Surgery

The Fundamentals of Laparoscopic Surgery (FLS) is a didactic and manual skills program designed to teach the basics of laparoscopic surgery to surgical trainees and surgeons. The training curriculum consists of 5 web-based modules and box-trainer self-practice of 5 surgical skills. Following this, individuals must undergo a 2-part proctored, standardized assessment that includes a technical and cognitive test of basic laparoscopic surgical skills.[24] The first assessment component is a web-based multiple choice examination, which focuses on intraoperative decision-making and clinical judgment. The second assessment consists of completion of 5 manual skills: peg transfer, precision cutting, placement/securing ligating loop, simple suture with extracorporeal knot, and simple suture with intracorporeal knot. These tests have substantial associated validity evidence and correspond well with a surgeon's ability to perform basic laparoscopic skills in the operating room.[25–28]

FLS is considered a high-stakes examination because passing both assessments is required by the ABS for graduating residents. It differs from other high-stakes examinations in that retakes are possible. If either or both assessments are failed, examinees must wait 30 days before retaking the failed portion of the assessment and must pay an additional retest fee. A second retest requires a 6-month hiatus before the examinations can be administered again.

### Fundamentals of Endoscopic Surgery

Similar to FLS, Fundamentals of Endoscopic Surgery (FES) is a teaching curriculum and a 2-part assessment developed by the Society of American Gastrointestinal and Endoscopic Surgeons. ABS has required surgical trainees to obtain FES certification before certification since 2018.[28] FES includes a teaching curriculum consisting of 12 web-based, interactive cognitive components and a 2-part assessment. The first is a 75 MCQ knowledge-based assessment that tests the clinical decision-making skills and appropriate application of upper and lower endoscopic techniques. The second is a proficiency-based assessment that tests speed and precision by measuring accuracy of the technical skills through 5 simulation exercises on the Simbionix laparoscopic simulator.[29] The tasks include navigation, loop reduction, targeting, mucosal evaluation, and retroflexion. These tasks test the psychomotor skills of the examinees and are graded based on speed and accuracy. Each of the 5 simulation cases is given the same weight. The content has been peer reviewed by surgeons and gastroenterologists and continues to be reviewed by the FES Test Committee for clinical relevance and psychometric evaluations to ensure that reasonable inferences can be made from the assessment score.

Validity evidence for the tests are substantial.[30,31] Assessment tools such as Global Assessment of Gastrointestinal Endoscopic Skills have been developed and used to demonstrate transferability of skills learned and assessed with FES to endoscopic procedures.[32] In addition, there is evidence to support that adding these standardized tests as a required part of ABS certification has strengthened the training of general surgery residents in these domains.[33]

### American Board of Surgery in Training Examination

Standardized testing during general surgery residency is most frequently encountered with American Board of Surgery in Training Examination (ABSITE). Although not required by the ABS, nearly all trainees take the test annually.

ABSITE is an MCQ examination consisting of 250 questions designed to assess residents' progress in clinically applied surgical knowledge and management of clinical problems related to surgery.[34] ABSITE is administered by programs across the United States as well as in 17 other countries. The ABSITE is the only standardized measure of resident knowledge that can be compared across training programs. It may also be useful in evaluation of individual program's education curriculum, as national comparative data are provided. Because the examination's results are only provided to the program directors, its intended purpose is as a needs assessment for learning. Good positive predictive value is demonstrated with ability to pass ABS board examinations.[9,35] However, the inverse has not been consistently true—lower scores do not necessarily predict failure. Intended as a low-stakes examination, the ABSITE provides a valuable tool for educators to identify and advise trainees who may benefit from focused instruction.[36] Program directors have reported using the ABSITE score as a factor in promotion of residents and also in identifying trainees who may be struggling with burnout or other wellness issues.[37,38] It remains unclear if ABSITE performance correlates with long-term clinical outcomes such as malpractice claims, restrictions on licensure, or complication rates. However, such associations do exist with ABS certification, and therefore, an inferred association may be appropriate.[39]

Despite the formative, low-stakes intention of the ABSITE, it has taken on some very high-stakes roles. It is widely used as a part of the fellowship selection process.[40–43] As such, it therefore takes on a similar purpose as the medical student NBME subject test in surgery in that performance can deter some residents from pursuing competitive specialties. Some residency programs also use the examination as a criterion to defer promotion of residents to the next training year.[37]

### American Board of Surgery—Qualifying and Certifying Examinations

The ABS qualifying examination (QE) and certifying examination (CE) are the standardized tests that allow a trainee to achieve board certification, a pivotal step in professional identity formation as a surgeon. ABS QE is the first in the series of 2 tests administered as a part of the general surgery board certification process. It consists of 300 MCQs that test knowledge pertinent to practicing general surgeons and application of this knowledge via "recall, synthesis, and judgment."[9] As the final step in the board certification process, ABS CE is an oral examination consisting of 3 consecutive half-hour sessions that assess the examinee's ability to efficiently and safely diagnose and manage surgical patients using applied clinical knowledge.

Given the enormous implications of board certification, the qualifying examination has been vetted through well-developed psychometrics[2]; this includes periodic review of content by the ABS directors and expert consultants. In addition, weighting of questions is assigned to emphasize topics relevant to clinical practice. Development of new questions and review of old questions that are vetted by specific committees occurs routinely. A combination of new and old questions with appropriate psychometric characteristics are included in the tests given to examinees.[9]

As high-stakes summative assessments, these tests are a focal point of studying and preparation throughout residency; this can create a paradox as to whether they are encouraging trainees to just learn the test or instead are an example of a well-designed assessment driving learning. In the case of the ABS examinations, the latter seems to be true, and this is evident in the effort the ABS has placed on not just creating the certification examinations but also collaborating with other organizations dedicated to surgical education to provide resources supporting attaining surgical knowledge and decision-making ability through the nonprofit Surgical Council on Resident Education.[44] With this collaboration a curriculum for graduate surgical education is available to guide educators and learners on the appropriate cognitive content necessary to train surgeons while also preparing them for testing.

### IDENTIFYING POTENTIAL AREAS FOR IMPROVEMENT

Although standardized tests are attractive as a way to assure a consistent measure of knowledge or skill, the potential for bias remains. A common statement among poor performers on standardized tests is that they are simply bad test takers. Although it is clear there is no set predisposition to specifically underperform on examinations, this may be related to test anxiety, learning disorders, and unintended cultural bias in addition to other factors.

### Emotional Stress

Test anxiety is a measurable phenomenon where information recall is suppressed by worry.[45] One might expect that this would not be an issue in graduate surgical education, given the high performance requirements on so many standardized tests to reach this level of training. However, poor preparation and low scores on examinations among medical students have been found associated with test anxiety.[46,47] Little has been written on the role of test anxiety on examination performance in surgical residency and beyond, but certainly an impact would be expected given its presence among medical students.

### Learning Disabilities

The prevalence of learning disabilities among surgical residents has not been described. However, around 3% of medical students have some form of identified disability, with attention deficit hyperactivity disorder and learning disabilities accounting for more than half of them.[48] It is therefore reasonable to presume that a population of learners in surgical training are affected by these. People with learning disabilities are afforded protection under the Americans with Disabilities Act.[49] The ABS complies with this law by allowing examinees to submit documentation of their need for testing accommodations. However, it is likely that many who have such disabilities may not disclose them to training programs or oversight bodies out of concern for implications on their professional standing; this is an area that warrants further investigation to mitigate stigma and bias.

### Bias

One of the most common unforeseen issues in standardized testing is bias. Biases have been documented in various standardized tests, and mitigation strategies must be a part of item creation to ensure fairness for all who take the examination.[50,51] Diverse groups of people should be involved in test creation and used as sample test takers, and the items should undergo DIF analysis. DIF is a subset of IRT used to determine if test scores differ between racial/ethnic groups, genders, social classes, etc.[52] For example, a standardized test could be deemed biased if white students were found to consistently score higher than Latinx students. Not only would the test items need to be reviewed for bias, the other testing materials and testing procedures would need to be scrutinized for fairness.[52] If a standardized test is deemed to be biased for or against a particular group of people, the test fails to adhere to its overall goal of measuring what the test is intended to measure.

Gender, cultural, and racial biases are present in most of the standardized tests required of surgical trainees. Psychometricians at the NBME demonstrated that test takers who are not native, English-speaking, white, male, US citizens of average age are likely to score lower on the USMLE examinations.[53] In the FES examination, men, who are taller and who have larger glove sizes, receive higher scores and pass more frequently.[54] Men are more likely to receive higher scores on the ABSITE.[55] White, non-Hispanic, examinees and women who were single at the time of their internship (compared with those who were unmarried with a partner, married with no children, or married with children at that time) are more likely to pass the ABS CE on their first attempt.[51] Mitigating these biases must be accomplished to assure standardized tests are actually achieving their intended outcomes.

## Cost

Financial requirements of standardized testing also contribute to the burden of these examinations in surgical training. Financial cost of the high-stakes ABS certification examinations alone cost trainees $1850 for QE and $1450 for CE in 2020 for examination registration alone.[56] This cost does not take into account travel and lodging necessary for CE. In addition, an industry has emerged for test preparation support, which also places financial strain on trainees. As requirements for board certification, examinations including FLS, FES, and ATLS, are often paid by the residency program and totaled $1530 in 2019.[57] FES has a high cost of implementation by testing centers estimated around $13,091 for personnel, equipment, and supplies.[58]

## LOOKING FORWARD

To address the gap in standardized tests available to assess intraoperative skills and surgical technique, research has shifted to evaluation of videos to assess intraoperative skills. Minimally invasive procedures including endoscopy, laparoscopic, and robotic surgeries can be conveniently recorded for assessment and review.[59] In the last decade, a growing number of research groups have conducted peer evaluation of intraoperative videos of laparoscopic bariatric procedures to identify near-miss events by using tool kits such as a modified version of Objective Structured Assessment of Technical Skill (OSATS) and Generic Error Rating Tool.[60,61] Birkmeyer and colleagues[60] demonstrated that peer review of a surgeon's skills correlated with the patient's clinical outcomes. One drawback for video-based assessment for trainees is inability to detect who was performing which segment of an operation. The ability to measure the learning curve of the trainees as they progress in training may also be important.[59]

Although an association has been shown between a surgeon's technical ability and their patient outcomes, few standardized tests of these skills exist.[62] The challenge of creating such a high-stakes examination is illustrated by the American Board of Colorectal Surgery's Colorectal Objective Structured Assessment of Technical Skill (COSATS).[63] This test included 8 skills assessed with individual task-specific checklists and a single global rating scale used together in scoring performance of each task. The test was successfully administered as a pilot and found to have appropriate evidence for validity across many domains.[64] It also was found to not correlate well with passage of the oral or written examination elements of board certification and therefore likely to assess a novel element of readiness for practice as a colorectal surgeon; this led to the creation of a similar model for general surgery, General Surgery Objective Structured Assessment of Technical Skill (GOSATS).[65] COSATS was not implemented as a requirement for board certification, though. The cost and effort of administering such an examination likely contributed to its lack of incorporation into the board certification process. In addition, questions remain about whether it is more appropriate to relegate an assessment of technical competence to standardized examinations such as these or to the judgment of program directors who have access to more extensive, longitudinal evaluations of trainee performance in this domain.

Limited standardized assessment of nontechnical skills (NTS) such as leadership, communication, professionalism, forward planning, teamwork, self-direction, patient safety, and situational awareness have been identified.[66] Although evaluation tools with validity evidence such as checklists and rating systems exist to assess NTS, standardization of these assessment tools is yet to be completed. Studies have demonstrated that poor nontechnical skills in the clinical settings can influence technical and subsequently patient outcome.[67] Early assessment of surgical trainees' NTS can prevent potential ABS certification failure because lacking NTS have been associated with failing ABS certification examinations.[68] Virtual reality (VR) simulators have gained increased footing in surgical education for surgical techniques and to a lesser degree for NTS. Although the possibility of using VR to teach learners NTS has been demonstrated, transfer of skills to real-life clinical scenarios have not been reported in current literature.[69] With ongoing advances in technology and its increasing presence in both surgical education and surgical management of patients, standardized assessment using advanced technology will greatly benefit surgical trainees.

## SUMMARY

Similar to other areas of medical education, standardized testing plays a valuable role in surgical education. High-stakes summative standardized tests for certification purposes serve to set the minimum benchmark for demonstration of surgical knowledge and skills expected from individual trainees. They also provide opportunity for comparison among trainees as well as of training programs. Formative standardized tests serve similar roles, but most importantly guide teaching endeavors for the programs and the individual trainees. They may also be used in applicant selection as an objective comparison among applicants. Ongoing rigorous psychometric evaluations of the standardized tests bolster their reliability. Evidence for test validity must be collected in as part of a continuous process. Identifying tests' limitations and mitigating biases is an important and active process. Endeavors in developing standardized testing to assess nontechnical skills and integration of new advances in technology will further improve the value of standardized testing in surgical education.

## DISCLOSURE

The authors have nothing to disclose.

## REFERENCES

1. About Us. Available at: http://www.absurgery.org/default.jsp?abouthome. Accessed October 1, 2020.
2. Frey B. The SAGE Encyclopedia of educational research, Measurement, and evaluation. 4th edition. Thousand Oaks (CA): SAGE Publications; 2018.
3. Yudkowsky R, Park YS, Downing S. Introduction to Assessment in Health Professions. In: Yudkowsky R, Park YS, Downing S, editors. Assessment in health Professions education. 2nd edition. London (UK): Routledge; 2019. p. 3–16.
4. Park YS. Reliability. In: Yudkowsky R, Park YS, Downing S, editors. Assessment in health Professions education. 2nd edition. London (UK): Routledge; 2020. p. 33–50.
5. Swanson DE, Hawkings RE. Using Written Examinations to Assess Medical Knowledge and Its Application. In: Holmboe E, Durning S, Hawkins R, editors. Practical guide to the evaluation of clinical competence. 2nd edition. Philadelphia: Elsevier; 2018. p. 113–39.
6. Park YS. Item Response Theory. In: Yudkowsky R, Park YS, Downing S, editors. Assessment in health Professions education. 2nd edition. London (UK): Routledge; 2020. p. 287–97.
7. Franzese CB, Stringer SP. The evolution of surgical training: perspectives on educational models from the past to the future. Otolaryngol Clin North Am 2007;40(6):1227–35, vii.

8. Epstein RM. Assessment in medical education. N Engl J Med 2007;356(20): 387–96.

9. Rhodes RS, Biester TW, Bell RH, et al. Assessing Surgical Knowledge: A Primer on the Examination Policies of the American Board of Surgery. J Surg Educ 2007; 64(3):138–42.

10. Ahmed A, Abid MA, Bhatti N. Balancing standardized testing with personalized training in surgery. Adv Med Educ Pract 2016;8:25–9.

11. National Board of Medical Examiners. Guide to the Subject Examination Program High-Quality Assessment Tools for Use in Medical Education Overview and Regulations for Use of Subject; 2020. Available at: https://www.nbme.org/sites/default/files/2020-01/subexaminfoguide.pdf. Accessed October 15, 2020.

12. Subject Examinations | NBME. Available at: https://www.nbme.org/assessment-products/assess-learn/subject-exams. Accessed November 2, 2020.

13. Schuman AD, Heisel CJ, Black KM, et al. Student Factors That Influence Clerkship Grades and Matching Into a Surgical Residency. J Surg Educ 2019;76(2): 393–400.

14. Awad SS, Liscum KR, Aoki N, et al. Does the subjective evaluation of medical student surgical knowledge correlate with written and oral exam performance? J Surg Res 2002;104(1):36–9.

15. American College of Surgeons and Association for Surgical Education. ACS/ASE Medical Student Core Curriculum. Available at: https://www.facs.org/education/program/core-curriculum. Accessed October 1, 2020.

16. American College of Surgeons. American College of Surgeons Entering Resident Readiness Assessment (ACS ERRA). Available at: www.facs.org/education/resources/acs-erra. Accessed July 15, 2020.

17. Sullivan ME, Park YS, Liscum K, et al. The American College of Surgeons Entering Resident Readiness Assessment Program. Ann Surg 2020;272(1): 194–8.

18. About Advanced Trauma Life Support. American College of Surgeons. Available at: https://www.facs.org/quality-programs/trauma/atls/about. Accessed October 28, 2020.

19. Booklet of Information - Surgery :22. Available at: American Board of Surgery, Booklet of Information https://www.absurgery.org/xfer/BookletofInfo-Surgery.pdf. Accessed October 15, 2020.

20. American College of Surgeons, Committee on Trauma. Advanced trauma life support, course administration and Faculty guide. 10th edition. Chicago (IL): American College of Surgeons; 2018.

21. Bustraan J, Henny W, Kortbeek JB, et al. MCQ tests in Advanced Trauma Life Support (ATLS©): Development and revision. Injury 2016;47(3):665–8.

22. Guido J, Telford B, Llerena LE, et al. The value of psychometric analysis of the advanced trauma life support cognitive test: Outcome of an ACS-Accredited educational institute multisite study. Am J Surg 2019;217(4):800–5.

23. Mobily M, Branco BC, Joseph B, et al. Predictors of failure in the Advanced Trauma Life Support course. Am J Surg 2015;210(5):942–6.

24. Fundamentals of Laparoscopic Surgery. Fundamentals of Laparoscopic Surgery. Available at: https://www.flsprogram.org/. Accessed October 1, 2020.

25. FLS Supporting Literature - Fundamentals of Laparoscopic Surgery. Available at: https://www.flsprogram.org/index/fls-supporting-literature/. Accessed November 2, 2020.

26. Zendejas B, Ruparel RK, Cook DA. Validity evidence for the Fundamentals of Laparoscopic Surgery (FLS) program as an assessment tool: a systematic review. Surg Endosc 2016;30(2):512–20.

27. Fried GM, Feldman LS, Vassiliou MC, et al. Proving the Value of Simulation in Laparoscopic Surgery. Ann Surg 2004;240(3):518–28.

28. Sturm LP, Windsor JA, Cosman PH, et al. A systematic review of skills transfer after surgical simulation training. Ann Surg 2008;248(2):166–79.

29. FAQ's. Fundamentals of Endoscopic Surgery. 2013. Available at: https://www.fesprogram.org/about/faqs/. Accessed November 2, 2020.

30. Vassiliou MC, Dunkin BJ, Fried GM, et al. Fundamentals of endoscopic surgery: creation and validation of the hands-on test. Surg Endosc 2014;28(3):704–11.

31. Poulose BK, Vassiliou MC, Dunkin BJ, et al. Fundamentals of Endoscopic Surgery cognitive examination: development and validity evidence. Surg Endosc 2014;28(2):631–8.

32. King N, Kunac A, Merchant AM. A Review of Endoscopic Simulation: Current Evidence on Simulators and Curricula. J Surg Educ 2016. https://doi.org/10.1016/j.jsurg.2015.09.001.

33. Weis JJ, Grubbs J, Scott DJ, et al. Are you better off than you were 4 years ago? Measuring the impact of the ABS flexible endoscopy curriculum. Surg Endosc 2020;34(9):4110–4.

34. Content Outline for the ABSITE®. :2. Available at: American Board of Surgery Content Outline for the ABSITE https://www.absurgery.org/xfer/GS-ITE.pdf. Accessed October 15, 2020.

35. Jones AT, Biester TW, Buyske J, et al. Using the American Board of Surgery In-Training Examination to Predict Board Certification: A Cautionary Study. J Surg Educ 2014;71(6):e144–8.

36. Cheun TJ, Davies MG. Improving ABSITE scores - A meta-analysis of reported remediation models. Am J Surg 2020. https://doi.org/10.1016/j.amjsurg.2020.04.028.

37. Taggarshe D, Mittal V. The Utility of the ABS In-Training Examination (ABSITE) Score Forms: Percent Correct and Percentile Score in the Assessment of Surgical Residents. J Surg Educ 2012;69(4):554–8.

38. Smeds MR, Thrush CR, McDaniel FK, et al. Relationships between study habits, burnout, and general surgery resident performance on the American Board of Surgery In-Training Examination. J Surg Res 2017;217:217–25.

39. Kopp JP, Ibáñez B, Jones AT, et al. Association Between American Board of Surgery Initial Certification and Risk of Receiving Severe Disciplinary Actions Against Medical Licenses. JAMA Surg 2020;155(5):e200093.

40. Miller AT, Swain GW, Widmar M, et al. How Important Are American Board of Surgery In-Training Examination Scores When Applying for Fellowships? J Surg Educ 2010;67(3):149–51.

41. Wach MM, Ayabe RI, Ruff SM, et al. A Survey of the Complex General Surgical Oncology Fellowship Programs Regarding Applicant Selection and Rank. Ann Surg Oncol 2019;26(9):2675–81.

42. Fraser JD, Aguayo P, St. Peter S, et al. Analysis of the pediatric surgery match: factors predicting outcome. Pediatr Surg Int 2011;27(11):1239–44.

43. Lam CC, Zimmern A. Colon and Rectal Surgery Residency Selection Criteria: A National Program Director Survey. J Surg Educ 2021. https://doi.org/10.1016/j.jsurg.2020.07.030.

44. SCORE | About SCORE. Available at: https://www.surgicalcore.org/public/aboutscore. Accessed October 1, 2020.

45. von der Embse N, Jester D, Roy D, et al. Test anxiety effects, predictors, and correlates: A 30-year meta-analytic review. J Affect Disord 2018;227:483–93.

46. Chapell MS, Blanding ZB, Silverstein ME, et al. Test Anxiety and Academic Performance in Undergraduate and Graduate Students. J Educ Psychol 2005;97(2): 268–74.

47. Powell DH. Behavioral treatment of debilitating test anxiety among medical students. J Clin Psychol 2004;60(8):853–65.

48. Meeks LM, Herzer KR. Prevalence of Self-Disclosed Disability Among Medical Students in U.S. Allopathic Medical Schools. JAMA 2016;316(21):2271–2.

49. Americans with Disabilities Act of 1990,AS AMENDED with ADA Amendments Act of 2008. Available at: https://www.ada.gov/pubs/adastatute08.htm. Accessed October 1, 2020.

50. Koenig JA, Sireci SG, Wiley A. Evaluating the Predictive Validity of MCAT Scores across Diverse Applicant Groups. Acad Med 1998;73(10):1095–106.

51. Yeo HL, Dolan PT, Mao J, et al. Association of Demographic and Program Factors With American Board of Surgery Qualifying and Certifying Examinations Pass Rates. JAMA Surg 2020;155(1):22.

52. Camilli G. Ongoing Issues in Test Fairness. Educ Res Eval 2013;19:104–20.

53. Rubright JD, Jodoin M, Barone MA. Examining Demographics, Prior Academic Performance, and United States Medical Licensing Examination Scores. Acad Med 2019;94(3):364–70.

54. Lineberry M, Matthew Ritter E. Psychometric properties of the Fundamentals of Endoscopic Surgery (FES) skills examination. Surg Endosc 2017;31(12): 5219–27.

55. Cassidy DJ, Chakraborty S, Panda N, et al. The Surgical Knowledge "Growth Curve": Predicting ABSITE Scores and Identifying "At-Risk" Residents. J Surg Educ 2020. https://doi.org/10.1016/j.jsurg.2020.06.038.

56. Dates and Fees - Training & Certification | American Board of Surgery. Available at: https://www.absurgery.org/default.jsp?examdeadlines. Accessed November 2, 2020.

57. Kempenich JW, Willis RE, Campi HD, et al. The Cost of Compliance: The Financial Burden of Fulfilling Accreditation Council for Graduate Medical Education and American Board of Surgery Requirements. J Surg Educ 2018;75(6):e47–53.

58. Nguyen PH, Acker CE, Heniford BT, et al. What is the cost associated with the implementation of the FLS program into a general surgery residency? Surg Endosc 2010;24(12):3216–20.

59. Loukas C. Video content analysis of surgical procedures. Surg Endosc 2018; 32(2):553–68.

60. Birkmeyer JD, Finks JF, O'Reilly A, et al. Surgical Skill and Complication Rates after Bariatric Surgery. N Engl J Med 2013;369(15):1434–42.

61. Bonrath EM, Gordon LE, Grantcharov TP. Characterising "near miss" events in complex laparoscopic surgery through video analysis. BMJ Qual Saf 2015; 24(8):516–21.

62. Stulberg JJ, Huang R, Kreutzer L, et al. Association Between Surgeon Technical Skills and Patient Outcomes. JAMA Surg 2020;155(10):960.

63. de Montbrun SL, Roberts PL, Lowry AC, et al. A Novel Approach to Assessing Technical Competence of Colorectal Surgery Residents: The Development and Evaluation of the Colorectal Objective Structured Assessment of Technical Skill (COSATS). Ann Surg 2013;258(6):1001–6.

64. de Montbrun S, Roberts PL, Satterthwaite L, et al. Implementing and Evaluating a National Certification Technical Skills Examination: The Colorectal Objective Structured Assessment of Technical Skill. Ann Surg 2016;264(1):1–6.

65. Halwani Y, Sachdeva AK, Satterthwaite L, et al. Development and evaluation of the General Surgery Objective Structured Assessment of Technical Skill (GO-SATS). BJS 2019;106(12):1617–22.

66. Sanfey H. Assessment of surgical training. Surgeon 2014;12(6):350–6.

67. Hull L, Arora S, Aggarwal R, et al. The impact of nontechnical skills on technical performance in surgery: a systematic review. J Am Coll Surg 2012. https://doi.org/10.1016/j.jamcollsurg.2011.10.016.

68. Dietl CA, Russell JC. Effects of Technological Advances in Surgical Education on Quantitative Outcomes From Residency Programs. J Surg Educ 2016;73(5):819–30.

69. Bracq M-S, Michinov E, Jannin P. Virtual Reality Simulation in Nontechnical Skills Training for Healthcare Professionals. Simul Healthc J Soc Simul Healthc 2019;14(3):188–94.

# Integration of Educational Technology

Aditi Jalla, MD, Jourdan Sturges, BS, Jason Lees, MD*

## KEYWORDS

- Database • Collaboration • Evaluation • Administrative • Platform • Organization
- Technology • Education

## KEY POINTS

- Education in its various forms requires organization and storage of materials as well as collaboration and delivery of content.
- Because of this very nature, utilization of technology continues to be a key aspect to all levels of education.
- This article outlines some aspects of integration of technology in mainstream education and showcases a few of the more frequently used services that are currently available.

## INTRODUCTION

In today's environment, it is impossible to administrate, organize, and deliver education without using technology. Medical educators are increasingly using technology to complement more traditional means of instruction. The continued evolvement of both the medical field and technology alike has resulted in unprecedented use of various online programs, databases, and tools. Each of these modalities endeavors to address different challenges that are faced within the medical academic community. Online administrative services seek to track and plan various programs and resident exercises that are required for accreditation. Other online services streamline delivery of documentation and learning materials. Conferencing applications allow effective, real-time communication without the inconvenience of in-person meetings. Mobile applications allow lecturers to engage their audience in the discussion in a simplified manner. Still, other online programs allow for easy communication between residents and the patients they are caring for. There is no question that technology will continue to advance at rapid rates; and as it develops, it will continue to take a leading role in our professional lives. For educators, the key is ensuring that each piece of technology is used in the most effective way possible. This article endeavors to explain how

University of Oklahoma Health Sciences Center College of Medicine, Department of Surgery, 800 SL Young Boulevard, Suite 9000, Oklahoma City, OK 73190, USA
* Corresponding author:
E-mail address: jason-lees@ouhsc.edu

Surg Clin N Am 101 (2021) 693–701
https://doi.org/10.1016/j.suc.2021.05.014
0039-6109/21/© 2021 Elsevier Inc. All rights reserved.

assorted technologies and online programs are currently used in surgical clinics across North America.

## ADMINISTRATIVE DATABASES

In order for residency programs to effectively manage their residents and faculty, they require organization through an administrative database. This organization can be multifaceted, including storage of basic personnel demographics and payroll details as well as a comprehensive human resources tool, allowing institutions to orchestrate processes such as onboarding and credentialing. The databases allow institutions to streamline these processes by addressing deadlines, creating automated reminders, and tracking progress. They also allow residents to manage their work schedules (on-call and rotation shifts, vacation requests, conference planning), assess individual performances, view performance evaluations, and track progress throughout training. For the institution, it permits program directors to review trainee hours and create customized goals for individuals. And on a more comprehensive scale, it allows institutional oversight by acting as a reporting engine, compiling all necessary documents across the program without the need for hours of data gathering; this is essential for accreditation and alumni management. Of course, these databases are not exclusive to graduate medical education but in fact are used by a wide variety of entities including undergraduate education, public and private corporations, and governmental bodies. Of the many available databases, a few are highlighted in the following section.

### Activity Insight

Activity Insight by Digital Measures/Watermark is an online system that is used by more than 500,000 medical faculty from across the nation.[1] This service enables residents and faculty to track their service, research, teach, and creative activities as they perform them. In addition, the program allows data from outside resources to be uploaded into the log to avoid redundancy of data collection, which allows residents to continuously keep their CVs updated in a single and secure location.[1]

### MedHub

MedHub is a Web-based administrative data hub that was designed specifically as a residency management system to simplify the interactions between a health system and its many resident programs. It was developed in 2002 by the Department of Surgery at the University of Michigan, and it was subsequently implemented in all 88 of University of Michigan's residency and fellowship programs in 2003.[2,3] Since then, MedHub has expanded to several hospitals, clinics, and universities across North America.

### New Innovations

New Innovations is a software-based Residency Management Suite that is similar to MedHub and caters to both Undergraduate Medical Education and Graduate Medical Education entities. Aside from similar services such as personnel management and streamlined onboarding and credentialing processes, New Innovations tracks each facility's accreditation process by focusing on compliance with the Accredition Council for Graduate Medical Education's Clinical Learning Environment Review program, which includes site visits. Facilities are able to send previsit surveys to residents to obtain informal opinions on compliance. Annual Program Evaluations grants programs the ability to create and distribute surveys while also permitting the creator to focus on specific areas by searching through "tags" in each evaluation; this allows directors to review strengths and weaknesses of their program in an efficient manner.[4]

## DELIVERY

In addition to administrative databases, there are management software systems designed primarily for content delivery. These systems are used to condense learning materials in an easily accessible location, record learners' progress through online assignments and quizzes, and catalog additional online resources for further learning.[5,6] Some systems foster creation of learning materials using their features, whereas others allow administrators to import materials from third-party services. In addition, they can allow direct communication between learners and educators as well as form-style discussions among classmates.

### Blackboard

Blackboard is a group of diverse learning and administration management systems that not only cater to higher education programs but also to other industries including K-12 education, government entities, and other businesses. Blackboard Learn is a learning management system that integrates course.

### Desire2learn

Founded in 1999 by engineering student John Baker, Desire2learn (D2L) is a widely used online learning system that is similar to Blackboard. D2L offers basic content utilization and delivery but also highlights video conferencing, personalized learning modules, online discussion forums, and completion certificates. These features allow for collaboration, commitment, communication, and motivation to each individual learner.[7–9] The Performance Plus add-on can be used as an analytics tool, which allows directors to generate data on individual performance and interpret predictive analytics. It can allow educators to customize the learning path for individual.

## VIDEO CONFERENCING

Although regular video conferencing has been the norm in several other industries, with the increase of the COVID-19 pandemic, education from elementary school to CME has been forced to incorporate video conferencing as a means to continue delivering and managing educational content in a safe and efficient manner. These applications allow multiple users to interact at once and allow them to experience "face-to-face" communication with options for sharing documents, broadcasting presentations, using chat features, and recording meetings. Users can broadcast lectures to viewers from anywhere in the world, allowing guest speakers to have more flexibility in terms of scheduling. Conversely, learners can also attend these virtual meetings from the comfort of home or from other remote locations, boosting attendance at such events. Institutions can choose from numerous options of video conferencing applications, each with various features. Ultimately, each institution and their IT department must assess the privacy requirements for their educational content and choose accordingly. Two of the most widely used video conferencing applications today are Google Meet (previously known as Google Hangouts) and Zoom (**Figs. 1** and **2**).

| | Skype | Google Hangouts | Proficonf | Appear.in | ZOOM | Uberconference | OOVOO | Jitsi Meet | Myownconference |
|---|---|---|---|---|---|---|---|---|---|
| Number of participants | up to 50 | up to 10 | up to 25 | up to 4 | up to 100 | up to 10 | up to 12 | unlimited | up to 20 |
| Storage capacity | ✓ | ✗ | 500 MB | ✗ | ✗ | ✗ | ✗ | ✗ | 500 MB |
| Video recording | ✓ * stored for up to 30 d | ✗ | ✗ | ✗ | ✓ up to 40 min | audio only | ✓ | ✓ * stored on your Dropbox | ✓ up to 20 min |
| Event duration | unlimited | unlimited | unlimited | unlimited | 40 min | 40 min | unlimited | unlimited | unlimited |
| No installation | ✗ | ✓ | ✓ | ✓ | ✗ | ✓ | ✗ | ✓ | ✓ |
| Support team | ✗ | ✗ | ✓ | ✓ | ✓ | ✓ | ✗ | ✗ | Mon-Sat, 9 a.m.-8p.m. |
| Screen demonstration | ✓ | ✗ | ✓ | ✓ | ✓ | ✓ | ✓ | ✗ | Flash Player extension |
| Presentation display capacity | ✗ | ✗ | ✓ | ✗ | ✗ | ✗ | ✗ | ✗ | ✗ |

**Fig. 1.** Proficonf. (*From* https://proficonf.com/ Original link: https://proficonf.com/the-9-best-video-conferencing-apps-in-2019/.)

## Google Meet

Google Meet, as other Google applications, interfaces with the company's various other applications such as Google Calendar and Google Docs. Functions provided by Google Meet include conferencing with or without video, screen sharing to display any relevant graphics, a messaging feature to encourage further conversation, and automatically generated captions to help everyone follow along with the discussion.[10,11] This application is used widely by educators from elementary schools to graduate colleges. In the health care fields, this application can be used to conduct video conferences to collaborate with other health care professionals from around the world and perform peer reviews.

## Zoom

Similar to Google Meet, Zoom is also emerging as a crucial aspect of continuing education during the pandemic. It offers comparable services and allows educators to deliver customized surveys to further engage their audience.[12] Zoom also interfaces with email and calendar applications and offers options for secure meetings that

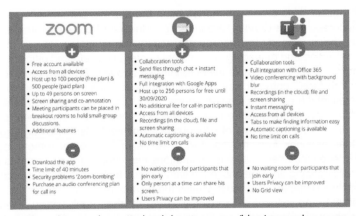

**Fig. 2.** Fourcast. (*From:* https://gcloud.devoteam.com/blog/comparing-zoom-microsoft-teams-and-google-meet.)

require not only the meeting link but 2 passwords as well. For health care educators, this is a useful tool that aids in Health Insurance Portability and Accountability Act (HIPAA) compliance.

### Audience Engagement

During live delivery of content, educators can assess audience engagement through real-time surveys and quizzes. There are several intranet and Internet applications that were already widely accepted by educators during in-person lectures; however, they are emerging as important tools in keeping audiences engaged during remote learning as well. Educators can open polls during their lectures and get instant feedback from their learners. In cases of difficult topics, teachers can adjust their presentation to accommodate for students struggling with the content. In addition, the more traditional route of preassessment and postassessment can be implemented to track progress made from the presentation. Directors can also ask open-ended questions to gain valuable insight or suggestions. This increases audience engagement and gives educators a sense of how their audience members are progressing in the learning process.

### Poll Everywhere

Poll Everywhere is a widely used Web-based polling application that allows presenters to engage with their audience through real-time questions and answers. It can be used to form contests and reports that provide knowledge to the physicians and residents of a clinic or hospital. In addition, users are given the right to anonymity, which can be advantageous when trying to establish honest feedback. Poll Everywhere questions can be embedded into presentations with PowerPoint, Google Slides, Keynote, and Slack; this allows educators to continue their presentations without having to switch to a different application, which allows for more streamlined content delivery. Similar to most audience engagement applications, Poll Everywhere can be used for in-person or remote learners.[13]

### Turning Technologies

Similar to Poll Everywhere, Turning Technologies has an interactive polling app called Turningpoint that can be used during presentations to enhance audience participation and engagement. Turningpoint can be used with any application using the floating toolbar feature that permits presenters to poll over the top of videos, presentations, Web pages, documents, or any other application that can be found on a desktop or mobile device.[14] The audience is able to answer prebuilt questions or those made up in the moment using either their mobile device or the Turning Technologies clicker. Anonymity is also an option with Turningpoint and allows for more authentic communication. Less traditional strategies can also be implemented using Turningpoint. Redsquare Audiovisuales, an AV company based in Spain, has used Turningpoint to create gamification within medical conferences across Spain. For example, they have incorporated Turningpoint into the presentations of Spanish Medical Society to create a Trivial Pursuit-like competition between attendees of the conference. They have used a similar strategy at other conferences wherein a medical debate takes place and the audience decides who moves forward in the "tournament" using polls from Turningpoint.[15] Similar to Poll Everywhere, the questions posed with Turningpoint during presentations can be used to encourage audience participation, thus improving the outcome of the discussion, generating communication between a presenter and his or her audience, and shaping future conversation based on feedback provided with the poll data.

## CLOUD-BASED STORAGE

Information management in the current technological age can be achieved through a variety of methods, one of which is cloud-based storage. This tool allows users to conveniently share data and make edits to documents, which can be visualized by all involved parties in real time, thus encouraging collaboration from any location. Cloud-based storage can be used to accumulate larger pieces of data, including journal articles, textbooks, and other learning materials that can be condensed into one location entirely online. Some cloud-based storage options provide a search function, thus drastically reducing the amount of time spent searching for specific information in a large document. In return, this information is accessible from any mobile or desktop device with an Internet connection.

### Google Docs

Google Drive is a cloud-based storage service that allows users to upload, share, and edit files within one location.[16] At the most basic level, Google Docs allows for the storage of up to 15 GB of free storage space, but more storage can be purchased with a set fee.[17,18] It is worth noting that following certain steps, it is possible to make Google Docs HIPAA compliant. In order to do so, entities must review and accept a Business Association Agreement (BAA). In addition, these entities must purchase G Suite Enterprise.[19] In doing so, Google will ensure that all documentation will have added protection. It is of worth to note that 100% compliance must be ensured by the user and cannot be completely fulfilled by the encryption and extra security put in place by the BAA and Google; this aids clinics and other health care facilities in using Google Docs for specific cases pertaining to patients.

### Microsoft OneDrive

Microsoft OneDrive is another cloud-based storage program that allows facilities and clinics to accumulate important documentation, textbooks, medical journals, and other learning materials in one account. In some cases, information can be shared with those outside of your own institution. For instance, those at Weill Cornell Medicine are able to share certain documents with peers from NYP, MSKCC, Rockefeller University, Cornell University, and many more.[20] In its most basic form, OneDrive offers 5 GB free storage to its users, and additional storage can be purchased for a set fee.[19] Furthermore, with selection of the "OneDrive for Business" plan, facilities are assured that they can use this service and still be compliant with HIPAA laws.[21]

## SURVEY AND DATA COLLECTION
### Qualtrics

Qualtrics is a Web-based survey program. In the medical world, clinics and facilities can use surveys to discern patient satisfaction with each of their experiences. These surveys can spotlight anything from their Web site experience, to any and every visit they have with physicians or staff, to specific points within the patient's journey in the clinic; this can include their satisfaction with their overall treatment or surgery. Examples of some of these prebuilt surveys include open heart surgery, joint replacements, or patient-reported outcomes. The Dashboard feature from Qualtrics allows its users to take data and transform it into reports, which can be shared with the rest of the facility. Examples of these prebuilt reports are inpatient experience, outpatient experience, overall customer experience, or how a specific location is meeting their internal goals. Physicians and clinics are then able to take the data supplied by these surveys and implement change within their own practice to better satisfy their patient base or better the overall patient outcome.[22–24] Perhaps the biggest benefit of Qualtrics is that physicians are quickly able to discover if their practice is being received in a positive light by their patients. Subsequently, they are able to rapidly take these insights and use them to alter or improve any aspect of their practice that is reflecting poorly on their facility or skills as a physician. In addition, the use of prebuilt surveys permits these physicians to spend more time with their actual patients as opposed to spending time with a computer screen while they create patient satisfaction surveys. Direct feedback from a patient serves as a helpful learning tool in ensuring that a provider or surgeon cares for his or her patient in the best way possible.

## REDCap

Entities involved in medical research have a keen interest in secure data collection, which necessitates a data collection system. One of the most widely used data collection systems is REDCap (Research Electronic Data Capture), a Web-based application developed at Vanderbilt University. REDCap not noly allows for simple data collection of sensitive data for clinical research projects but it also allows certain users with specific permission to export the information for statistical analysis. Administrators can use REDCap to generate surveys, capture electronic signatures, and create various types of questions for their project. Uses of this software include data collection for Institutional Review Board studies, information capture from electronic health records, generating surveys to send to patients, quality improvement studies, and more.[25] Specifically, surgical clinics across North America have used REDCap to investigate outcomes of elective orthopedic surgeries, implement an RAI-Frailty Screening for a vascular surgery clinic in the southwest, and manage many other preoperative and postoperative projects, studies, and surveys.[26,27] Any enterprise that requires the compilation of sensitive data can benefit from the use of a secure data collection application such as REDCap.

## SUMMARY

Overall, technological options for the collection, distribution, and interaction of educational content are abundant and versatile. Most of the aforementioned modalities of educational technology are accompanied by mobile applications, which allow for even more convenient access to the content. This chapter provides a general overview of available technologies and is by no means an exhaustive list of systems. Ultimately, in deciding the best options, specific entities will need to not only assess their platform needs but also ensure compliance with their specific institutional policies. And of course, as is standard with technology, the only certainty is that currently available technologies will change and may even become obsolete in a short amount of time.

## DISCLOSURE

The authors have nothing to disclose.

## REFERENCES

1. Opsa.siu.edu. 2020 [online] Available at: https://ospa.siu.edu/_common/documents/faculty-guidance-on-use-of-activity-insight.pdf. Accessed November 15, 2020.
2. MedHub. University of Michigan Health System Case Study – Medhub. 2020 [online] Available at: https://www.medhub.com/customers/success-stories/university-of-michigan-health-case-study/. Accessed November 15, 2020.

3. MedHub. GME Features Overview – Medhub. 2020 [online] Available at: https://www.medhub.com/software-solutions/gme/features/. Accessed November 15, 2020.

4. Innovations, N.. New Innovations – GME. 2020 [online] Available at: https://www.new-innov.com/pub/gme.html. Accessed November 15, 2020.

5. D2L. About Us|D2L. 2020 [online] Available at: https://www.d2l.com/about/. Accessed November 15, 2020.

6. Scranton.edu. Desire2learn Learning Management System | Information Technology. 2020 [online] Available at: https://www.scranton.edu/information-technology/services/lms.shtml#:%7E:text=Desire2Learn%20(D2L)%20is%20a%20web,online%20and%20around%20the%20world.%26text=Organizes%20e%2Dlearning%20materials%20in,access%20to%20e%2Dlearning%20materials. Accessed November 15, 2020.

7. D2L. Brightspace Core for Corporate |Engaging Learning Experience |Brightspace By D2L. 2020 [online] Available at: https://www.d2l.com/corporate/products/core/. Accessed November 15, 2020.

8. D2L. Learning Analytics Software |Brightspace by D2L. 2020 [online] Available at: https://www.d2l.com/corporate/products/performance/. Accessed November 15, 2020.

9. Zoom Video. Video Conferencing, Web Conferencing, Webinars, Screen Sharing. 2020 [online] Available at: https://zoom.us/about. Accessed November 15, 2020.

10. Workspace.google.com. Google Workspace – Collaboration Software for Healthcare. 2020 [online] Available at: https://workspace.google.com/industries/healthcare/. Accessed November 16, 2020.

11. Poll Everywhere. Poll Everywhere for Healthcare Systems. 2020 [online] Available at: https://www.polleverywhere.com/healthcare-systems. Accessed November 16, 2020.

12. Zoom.us. 2020 [online] Available at: https://zoom.us/docs/doc/Video%20Communications%20in%20Healthcare.pdf. Accessed November 15, 2020.

13. Poll Everywhere. Poll Everywhere Applications. 2020 [online] Available at: https://www.polleverywhere.com/app. Accessed November 16, 2020.

14. Turning Technologies. Anywhere Polling: Add Interactive Questions Anytime, Anywhere|Turning Technologies. 2020 [online] Available at: https://www.turningtechnologies.com/news-and-events/tips/anywhere-polling-add-interactive-questions-anytime-anywhere/. Accessed November 17, 2020.

15. Turning Technologies. Using Audience Response Systems to Train 21st Century Medical Students|Turning Technologies. 2020 [online] Available at: https://www.turningtechnologies.com/news-and-events/tips/using-audience-response-systems-to-train-21st-century-medical-students/. Accessed November 17, 2020.

16. Ventola C. Mobile Devices and Apps for Health Care Professionals: Uses and Benefits. 2020 [online] PubMed Central (PMC). Available at: https://www.ncbi.nlm.nih.gov/pmc/articles/PMC4029126/. Accessed November 17, 2020.

17. GeeksforGeeks. Difference Between Microsoft Onedrive and Google Drive – Geeksforgeeks, . . [online] Available at: https://www.geeksforgeeks.org/difference-between-microsoft-onedrive-and-google-drive/. Accessed November 17, 2020.

18. Anna Luan M. Cloud-Based Applications for Organizing and Reviewing Plastic Surgery Content. 2020 [online] PubMed Central (PMC). Available at: https://www.ncbi.nlm.nih.gov/pmc/articles/PMC4644353/. Accessed November 17, 2020.

19. HIPAA Guide. Is Google Docs HIPAA Compliant? – HIPAA Guide. 2020 [online] Available at: https://www.hipaaguide.net/is-google-docs-hipaa-compliant/. Accessed November 17, 2020.
20. Its.weill.cornell.edu. Onedrive Cloud Storage – Beta|Information Technologies & Services. 2020 [online] Available at: https://its.weill.cornell.edu/services/online-collaboration-storage-servers/onedrive-cloud-storage-beta. Accessed November 17, 2020.
21. Niedig S. *Is Microsoft Onedrive HIPAA Compliant? |Gazelle Consulting.* 2020 [online] Gazelle Consulting. Available at: https://gazelleconsulting.org/is-onedrive-hipaa-compliant/. Accessed November 17, 2020.
22. Qualtrics. Patient Customer Experience|Qualtrics. 2020 [online] Available at: https://www.qualtrics.com/marketplace/patient-experience/. Accessed November 17, 2020.
23. Image. Available at: https://www.fourcast.io/blog/comparing-zoom-microsoft-teams-and-google-meet.
24. Image. Available at: https://proficonf.com/the-9-best-video-conferencing-apps-in-2019/.
25. Partridge E, Bardyn T. Research Electronic Data Capture (REDCap). Journal of Medical Library Association. Available at: https://www.ncbi.nlm.nih.gov/pmc/articles/PMC5764586/. Accessed November 17, 2020.
26. Piuzzi N, Strnad G, Brooks P, et al. Implementing a Scientifically Valid, Cost-Effective and Scalable Data Collection System at Point of Care (The Cleveland Clinic OME Cohort). J Bone Joint Surg 2019 [online] Available at: https://pubmed.ncbi.nlm.nih.gov/30845040/. Accessed November 17, 2020.
27. Tucker P, Flink B, Varley P, et al. Implementation of A RAI-Frailty Screening Across Surgical Clinics: A Quality Improvement Initiative. 2016 [online] Available at: https://qualitysafety.bmj.com/content/25/12/1012.1. Accessed November 17, 2020.

# Continuing Medical Education and Lifelong Learning

Callie D. McAdams, MD, Michael M. McNally, MD*

## KEYWORDS

- Education • Coaching • Simulation • Competency • CPD • MOC • PBLI • CME

## KEY POINTS

- Continuing medical education is a broadly defined educational process that assists physicians in completing their professional responsibilities in a more effective and efficient manner.
- Maintenance of certification has 4 components: professional standing; lifelong learning and self-assessment; assessment of knowledge, judgment, and skills; and improvement in medical practice. These components are derived from the American College of Graduate Medical Education 6 core competencies to exemplify a competent physician.
- Lifelong learning is a continuous process where the learners gains knowledge and skills through peer support to be applied to their practice. Examples of lifelong learning include simulation, coaching, and communities of practice.
- Continuous professional development is a comprehensive educational design that is individualized, learner centered, and focused on numerous professional education facets.

## INTRODUCTION

In the rapidly changing world of health care, providers are encouraged and often required to keep up to date with education to deliver excellent patient care. During residency, acquisition of skills and education is highly structured, which guides learners to ultimately become competent surgeons.[1] After residency, learning is more nebulous, requiring learners to navigate the process of keeping competence while balancing clinical and administrative duties. Previously concerns were raised about the adequacy of physician training and ultimately the safety of patients.[2] It has been proved that a decrease in factual knowledge worsens with time, and reviews found that physicians that practiced for longer periods of time may have worse patient outcomes.[3] From these concerns, guidelines and programs were developed to establish a maintenance of certification (MOC) for physicians.[4]

Division of Vascular Surgery, Department of Surgery, University of Tennessee, 1940 Alcoa Highway, Building E, Suite 120, Knoxville, TN 37920, USA
* Corresponding author.
E-mail address: mmcnally@utmck.edu

Surg Clin N Am 101 (2021) 703–715
https://doi.org/10.1016/j.suc.2021.05.015
0039-6109/21/© 2021 Elsevier Inc. All rights reserved.

In 1933, several established medical boards, along with the American Medical Association's Council on Medical Education, the Federation of State Medical Boards, Association of American Medical Colleges, and American Hospital Association coalesced to form the Advisory Board of Medical Specialties. The Advisory Board of Medical Specialists was renamed in 1970 to the current American Board of Medical Specialties (ABMS).[5] This board encompasses multiple specialties across medicine and sets the standards for certification. In 2020, the ABMS issued certifications for 40 general specialties and 87 subspecialities and certifies more than 900,000 physicians currently.[6] The American Board of Surgery joined this association in 1937.[7] Although each specialty is under the ABMS, the individual specialty boards are responsible for creating content that completes the requirements set forth by the ABMS.[5]

This article reviews the development of the 6 core competencies, MOC, lifelong learning, and continuous professional development (CPD), and how each one affects surgical education for practicing physicians.

## AMERICAN COLLEGE OF GRADUATE MEDICAL EDUCATION 6 CORE COMPETENCIES

In 1999, the American College of Graduate Medical Education (ACGME) created the 6 core competencies and subsequently launched the Outcomes Project in 2001.[8] The 6 core competencies are medical knowledge, patient care, interpersonal and communicative skills, professionalism, practice-based learning and improvement (PBLI), and systems-based practice. These competencies were initially developed to accomplish the goal of creating a competency-based medical education model, which had been developed in academic fields other than medicine.[9] This style of education in its purest form allows learners to advance through material as they are able and provides additional time to those who needed it.[10] In the setting of medical education, medical graduates may be older and have restricted work hours that make the previous master-apprentice or random-encounters model of medical learning inadequate.[11,12] To fulfill both needs, a hybrid approach was developed that uses competency milestones and frequent assessments, all within the time constraints for medical education and training.[8]

Although the 6 core competencies were originally developed for medical education, they became a standard for all health care workers.[13] The ABMS also identified the same 6 core competencies as standards for practicing surgeons.[1,8] Although these 6 competencies are all important, the dedicated time and weight assigned to each competency changes over time.[1] In early education and residency training, the core of medical knowledge and patient care typically are emphasized more heavily. All physicians, whether training or practicing, should have educational activities centered on the competencies of interpersonal and communication skills and professionalism. However, for practicing surgeons, more time should be dedicated to PBLI and systems-based practice.[1]

PBLI as a core competency is a cycle that allows physicians to learn and develop from previous experiences.[14] If used correctly and practiced in residency, it provides a framework for future learning and growth. This competency involves 4 steps: identifying areas for improvement, engaging in learning, applying the new knowledge and skills to practice, and checking for improvement.[15] PBLI is never truly finished, but instead continues increasing in complexity as the surgeon grows.

The first step of identifying areas for improvement is crucial for initiating the PBLI cycle. In particular with self-assessment, identification of improvement areas can be difficult for surgeons. Research has shown that self-assessment is often ineffective and fails to identify true gaps in knowledge. In addition, the worst correlations in self-assessment have been found in physicians who are the least skilled or most confident.[16] One way to standardize the process and evaluate for areas for improvement is through outcome-based reflection, either by using local outcomes data or participating in a registry such as the National Surgical Quality Improvement Program (NSQIP).[14] This method allows surgeons to compare outcomes of their procedures with those of their peers and identify gaps for improvement.

Step 2 of the PBLI process is engaging in learning. During medical school and residency, this is highly structured but, during practice, physicians must balance this with other duties of practice. This material should be specific to the education gap identified in step one of the PBLI process. The learning material in this process can be varied, including traditional didactic lectures, case studies, or simulation courses to develop new surgical skills.[14,15]

Step 3 of applying new knowledge and skills can be a difficult process for physicians to perform, especially if the physician struggles with self-assessment. Preceptors and mentors are particularly helpful for implementing new skills into practice.[14,17] Surgical coaches can also help physicians implement a new technical skill and give directed feedback. The coaching feedback can happen electronically using video recording and teleproctoring or it can happen in person at the physician's institution.[14]

The final step in the PBLI process is checking for improvement. Improvements in knowledge can be assessed using examinations or case-based scenarios for decision making.[15] New surgical skills or procedures can be examined with simulation or review of procedure outcomes.[14] Proctors can be used to assess surgeons' skills and report feedback to the physicians.[17] Communication skills also can be assessed by using 360 evaluations, which provide feedback from an entire health care team.[15] As physicians check for improvement, they can identify additional areas for improvement and then the cycle restarts. PBLI, along with the other 6 core competencies, sets the framework for all forms of continuing medical education (CME) for practicing surgeons.

## MAINTENANCE OF CERTIFICATION

Initially certification was a lifelong designation without any additional requirements. In the 1970s, individual boards began limiting their certification length, requiring members to recertify every 6 to 10 years,[18] which resulted in the development of the MOC program, which is continually refined. In 2020, the ABMS released their recommendations from the Vision Initiative Commission, which contained 14 goals to continue to improve the certification processes for physicians.[19]

MOC has 4 components: professional standing; lifelong learning and self-assessment; assessment of knowledge, judgment, and skills; and improvement in medical practice. Each component has several subcomponents to be addressed. These components are derived from the 6 core competencies to exemplify a competent physician set forth by the ACGME and ABMS.

Professional standing simply requires that a physician hold a current medical license.[20] Previously, lapses or loss of licensure would preclude certification, but the 2014 standards for MOC set forth by the ABMS require boards to have processes in place for examining the circumstances surrounding licensure and weigh them appropriately.[21] Each board requires different additional components to prove professional standing. For example, the American Board of Surgery also requires letters of reference for professionalism and a 12-month operative log for physicians that hold operative credentials at a hospital.[22]

Lifelong learning and self-assessment address the needs of maintaining a knowledge base, which is attained through CME credits. These credits address general topics but can be tailored to individual practice needs. These CME credits can also be on nonclinical topics, including quality improvement, professionalism, and ethics.[6,23] In additional to CME credits, some boards require a self-assessment to be performed in conjunction with CME. These self-assessment modules (SAMs) were initially designed to allow physician reflection during the education session.[20] SAMs are not meant to be punitive, and incorrectly answering questions does not necessarily disqualify the learner. SAMs are administered after specific lectures or readings or can be globally comprehensive. For example, a comprehensive SAM is the Surgical Education and Self-Assessment Program provided by the American College of Surgeons.[22] SAMs take many forms, including interactive questions during lectures, postlecture posttests, or online questionnaires.[20] The number of SAMs required for MOC varies among different specialties, with some boards not requiring them at all.[20,24]

Assessment of knowledge, judgment, and skills, formerly named cognitive expertise, involves examination of the core content, judgment, and skills within a field.[5] Per the ABMS, this examination must be performed at a minimum every 10 years.[6] The type of examination is left to the individual boards. These MOC examinations require safeguards to verify that the physician recertifying is truly the test taker, examination content is not distributed among other test-takers, and materials used during the examination are approved by the ABMS.[6] The approach to this examination is different among specialties. Some use traditional high-stakes in-person examinations, whereas others allow shorter examinations with the ability to use resources during the examination.[5,24]

Improvement in medical practice entails any activity that engages the physicians to critically evaluate their skills and patient outcomes. Such activities may include patient logs, participation in registries, quality improvement data, practice improvement modules, or patient surveys.[14,22] Some surgical examples include participation in the NSQIP or National Trauma Database for level I and II trauma centers.[22] Improvement in medical practice can also be applied to multidisciplinary teams to improve the health care system.[5,6,20]

MOC was always meant to be an elective pursuit for physicians and not a minimum standard. Studies have been performed to analyze whether maintaining certification translates to professional behavior. A study performed in 2018 analyzed certification and loss-of-license actions in American Board of Surgery (ABS)–certified general surgeons.[25] This study analyzed more than 15,000 surgeons divided into 3 groups (on-time recertification, lapsed recertification, and not-recertified status) and then compared the groups with loss-of-license actions. Surgeons in the on-time recertification group had the lowest rate of loss of license, compared with both the lapsed recertification and not-recertified groups. Although this study does not determine causality, it did show that there was a correlation between maintaining certification in a timely manner and licensure actions.[25]

Attitudes to MOC have been studied and the results have been mixed. A small study was performed by Bower and colleagues[26], of physicians of all types within the state of Oregon concerning maintaining certification. Participants were asked whether they planned on recertifying and, if so, what their reasons were for pursuing recertification. Of the respondents to the survey, 95% of physicians with time-limited certifications planned to recertify and 12% of those with lifetime certifications planned to recertify voluntarily. Assessment of the motivations for this study group found that most physicians were pursing recertification to show that expertise, competency, or medical knowledge in their field was up to date.[26] Fewer physicians reported that their motivations were hospital or group practice requirements. The physicians who participated were asked about which resources were provided to them for help with recertification. Only 32% were provided time off from practice to pursue MOC and only 36% had financial support; 29% reported no resources provided from their practice groups. Although this study shows that most motivations are positive and intrinsic, there is still a disconnect on how to support physicians through the certification process.[26]

A secondary analysis was performed of the participants in the Bower and colleagues[27] study of physicians in Oregon, evaluating the physician preferences to CME. Many physicians that participated preferred traditional types of CME (conferences, review courses, and journals), with the favorite being medical association meetings. Individual training sessions or computer-based education was the least preferred. In addition, physicians preferred more passive forms of education, particularly large group lectures rather than individualized or small group sessions. Physicians were clustered within the study by type of physician. Overall, academic physicians were less likely to prefer innovative forms of CME rather than mostly clinical physicians.[27] Few of the physicians surveyed were interested in courses on quality improvement, communication, or professionalism,[27] which are 3 of the 6 core competencies.[8] Bower and colleagues[27] hypothesized that physicians are comfortable with traditional learning methods from the years of success in undergraduate and graduate courses using the same models. Low physician interest in nontraditional education formats has stymied CME innovation and stands as a challenging opportunity to develop nontraditional CME that appeals to providers.[27]

Although there are barriers to MOC for physicians, elimination of most of these barriers does not ensure use of MOC education. For example, the University of North Carolina level I trauma center is the leader of their region in trauma. They hosted an American College of Surgeons' Committee on Trauma course, named Rural Trauma Team Development, which was relevant to the mostly rural region served by the University of North Carolina. The regional course was available for all physicians and other health care providers of a multidisciplinary trauma team. The course was 1 day in length and free of charge to all recipients. Over the course of 3 years, 22 courses were offered and a total of 234 trauma care providers attended. However, only 7.7% of providers that attended were physicians and none of them were surgeons. This absence was noted by other nonphysician attendees. Postcourse surveys often stated that the lack of attendance by surgeons created concerns that they would be unable to translate what they had learned in the course to practice without the participation of physicians in the course.[28] Despite these courses being offered locally and free of charge, two of the largest barriers to participating in CME, this course shows the disconnect between those providing CME and the learners themselves. These studies show the need to develop CME that is appealing to physicians to encourage participation.

## AMERICAN BOARD OF SURGERY AND CONTINUOUS CERTIFICATION

Previously the ABS required an initial certification comprising a 2-step process requiring a written examination followed by an oral examination.[28] A recertification examination was then required every 10 years. This reexamination was an in-person, high-stakes examination and often required physicians to travel and leave their practice duties.[29] In addition, the second component of MOC, lifelong learning and self-assessment, was fulfilled by accumulating 150 American Medical Association Physician's Recognition Award category 1 credits, with 50 of these being self-assessment credits in a 5-year period.[15] This burden was reported as being significant to practicing surgeons. In 2017, the ABS performed a survey concerning MOC and examinations. Of the almost 10,000 diplomates that responded, 80% thought that examination material should be focused on the core principals of surgery and be related to their practice.[30] Sixty percent of the survey participants expressed that they would prefer the high-stakes, 10-year examination to be replaced with a more frequent examination that would be open book. Only 13% of respondents were still in favor of the 10-year examination. Sixty-seven percent of respondents thought that the optimum testing interval for examination would be every 2 years.[30] In response to these results, the ABS undertook a significant change.

In 2018, the ABS changed their MOC program and renamed it the Continuous Certification Program.[29] With this update came a change in examinations and continuous knowledge. The program began enrolling diplomates whose certification would expire in 2019. The previous 10-year examination was replaced with an examination that would be performed every 2 years. The new examination is significantly shorter, consisting of only 40 questions. Twenty questions involve core surgery and 20 questions are practice related. The practice-related areas are chosen by the diplomate and include comprehensive general, abdomen, alimentary tract, or breast surgery.[29] This examination is computerized and may be taken wherever the diplomate chooses. Once started, the test taker has 2 weeks to complete the assessment and may save the examination at any time. It is an open-book test and all content is published in advance on the ABS Web site.[24] The test taker gets immediate feedback and 2 attempts to answer correctly. Ultimately a score of 80% is required to pass, but a second attempt is granted if 40% is achieved on the first examination.[24] If test takers are unable to pass their second attempts by 80%, they enter a grace year period, which does not affect their certification.[31]

The other requirements for the Continuous Certification Program have changed as well. The CME credit requirements decreased. After passing the first examination, diplomates are only required to fulfill 125 category 1 CME credits and no self-assessment component is required.[24] Diplomates are required to keep a valid, unrestricted state medical license and have surgical privileges if still clinically working. Diplomates must complete a 12-month operative experience report every 10 years and have 2 professional reference forms submitted every 5 years. Surgeons must participate in a local, regional, or national outcomes registry or quality assessment program to fulfill the fourth requirement of MOC, improvement in medical practice.[24] The Continuous Certification Program culminates in a much more holistic and practical program for practicing surgeons, requiring less time to prepare for examinations, decreased anxiety, and no need to leave a practice for examinations.

## LIFELONG LEARNING

Lifelong learning is important for surgeons to provide safe, up-to-date care. Lifelong learning is a continuous process where the learners gain knowledge and skills through peer support to be applied to their practice.[32] Lifelong learning is different than the learning of undergraduate students, medical students, and residents. As opposed to the short time spent in formal education, physicians spend multiple decades as practicing physicians, making lifelong learning crucial for safe patient care.[17,33]

Motivation of the physician plays heavily into lifelong learning. Under the self-determination theory of motivation, there are sources of autonomous motivation (AM) and controlled motivation (CM).[34] AM is associated with intrinsic motivating factors and typically a longer-lasting, positive type of motivation. CM is associated with extrinsic sources of motivation, such as an incentivized reward or punishment avoidance. With CM, motivating factors are shorter lasting and more negative.[34] In a 2018 study, physicians in the Netherlands were surveyed to identify their motivational profiles.[35] The study found female physicians were more likely to have a high degree of AM than their male counterparts. Physicians in surgical specialties were more likely to have a high degree of AM. Interestingly, the age of the physician and length of practice negatively correlated with motivation, and these groups were more likely to have less AM and more CM factors. Because it is well known that motivation for lifelong learning is associated with more AM, the program developers should understand the underlying motivations of their audience and try to develop environments that stimulate each learner.[35]

## LIFELONG LEARNING THROUGHOUT SURGEONS' CAREERS

Lifelong learning changes as surgeons advance through their careers. Sachdeva and colleagues[17] divide surgeons' careers into 3 main sections: entry into practice, core professional practice, and transition out of practice. Entry into practice focuses on the first 2 to 3 years out of residency as the surgeon is starting to practice. Here the main goal is to establish that the surgeon is safe and competent to practice. Preceptorship and simulation can be used to ensure that the surgeon is safe to perform procedures. During this initial period, there may be a sign-off process to ensure competence in surgical skills.[17] Preceptors can also help new surgeons navigate difficult clinical decisions and complex patients. Core professional practice is the second phase of a surgeon's career, which encompasses the 20 to 30 years that surgeons practice. Acquisition of new skills as technology advances and the mastery of skills are crucial.[17] In this phase of the physician's career, problem-based learning and improvement is key for physicians to identify knowledge gaps and address them.[36] Simulation and coaching can be used to introduce new skills. Morbidity and mortality conferences can lead to individual and systems improvements. Practice or skill development–designed courses can promote mastery of skills.[17] The final phase of each surgeon's career is the transition out of practice. As senior surgeons reduce their clinical workloads, they are ideal candidates to serve as the mentors, coaches, and preceptors needed for practicing surgeons.[12,17]

Reentry into practice is another area of lifelong learning within physicians' careers. Physicians may exit the field for personal or family reasons, pursue administrative or nonclinical duties, or take time for a sabbatical.[17] If these individuals decide to reenter clinical practice, there are different platforms to provide a support system in place to help ease their reentry to practice. Examples include structured preceptorship or simulation to ensure the physician's surgical skills are adequate.[17,36,37] Certifying boards may also have criteria that need to be met before physicians can reenter clinical practice.[36]

Lifelong learning encompasses many different components, including but not limited to simulation, coaching, quality improvement through mortality and morbidity (M&M) conferences, professional courses, and communities of practice.

## SIMULATION

Simulation is an excellent tool for physicians to continue to improve technical and nontechnical skills. Although the use of simulation for residents is well known, including examinations such as the Fundamental Skills of Laparoscopic Surgery and Fundamentals of Endoscopic Surgery,[38] the use of simulation in lifelong learning can be beneficial. Simulation provides an area for physicians to safely reflect on clinical decisions and errors in a nonpunitive manner.[39] In 2005, the American College of

Surgeons developed the American College of Surgeons Accredited Education Institutes (ACS-AEIs).[40] ACS-AEIs is a system for simulation centers across America to become accredited as either a level I or level II center.[37] These centers provide a wide variety of simulations for physicians to learn from standardized patients, tasks simulators, or computer-based simulations. The courses they offer can also be nontechnical, including cognitive, professionalism, or communication simulation.[37,39] ACS-AEIs allow physicians to learn new skills or practice infrequently performed procedures in a safe environment. In addition, the accreditation process ensures that physicians across the country have access to high-quality, verified simulation education.[40]

## SURGICAL COACHING

Surgical coaching is a useful tool for maintaining and improving surgical skills in practice. Coaching within surgery can be used for a variety of technical, nontechnical, and cognitive skills.[41] These sessions should be structured and allow for self-assessment, goal setting, guidance, and feedback.[41,42] Coaching can be performed in person or remotely via recorded videos of surgical procedures.[42–44] In a 2019 review article, surgical coaching was used to help transfer skills, both technical and nontechnical, to middle-income and low-income countries to help improve global surgery.[42] In addition, systematic reviews have proved that coaching improves surgical skills, knowledge, and satisfaction scores among learners.[45]

Coaching is more structured than experiential learning. In a single-institution study, residents were randomized to either conventional residency training or comprehensive surgical coaching.[44] Surgical coaching involved debriefing of a previously recorded procedure and developed strategies to improve the technical difficulties within the procedure.[44] After 2 months of training, objective assessments of technical skills were performed and the residents within the coaching group performed better technically than the conventional group. Interestingly, a secondary outcome of this study showed that the residents who had coaching had self-assessment scores that correlated correctly with their level of technical skill, as opposed to the conventional group.[44]

Coaching is useful outside the scope of residency. In Wisconsin, a peer coaching program was developed to allow practicing physicians to match with coaches throughout the state on both technical and nontechnical aspects of surgery.[43] Participants prerecorded videos of themselves performing procedures and met with coaches for approximately 1 hour in person. Evaluation from the program found that participants found the sessions highly valuable and were satisfied with their experiences. Although most participants stated that their main objective for pursuing coaching was to improve a technical skill, less than half of the participants focused solely on their main objectives. Most participants also wanted to discuss the interpersonal, cognitive, and stress management portions of their intraoperative videos.[43] This finding further shows the usefulness of coaching as a tool for lifelong learning and professional development.

## MORBIDITY AND MORTALITY CONFERENCES

M&M conferences are used by residency programs to fulfill 2 of the 6 core competencies set forth by the ACGME: practice-based learning improvement and systems-based practice.[4] They provide a forum for individual cases to be analyzed and to evaluate patient outcomes. Practicing surgeons can use M&M conferences to identify areas of concern in their own practice. The act of preparing conference, presenting cases, and creating goals for change is beneficial to practicing surgeons.[17] Multidisciplinary M&M conferences have changed from assigning blame to individual practitioners to assessing where errors occur within the system of health care that can be addressed with quality improvement projects.[4]

A study performed by Lei and colleagues[46] in 2017 examined physician behavior after participating in a surgical audit in Queensland, Australia. As part of CPD, physicians must participate in the Queensland Audit of Surgical Mortality (QASM). Surgeons may submit cases for evaluation or be an assessor of mortality cases. Physicians who participated were given a survey to elucidate whether participation in QASM had changed their surgical practice. The study showed that 39% of surgeons changed their clinical practice and 19% thought that it affected their hospital practice.[46] Open-ended responses from participants showed they felt more confident using best-practice methods, thought their communication with documentation improved, and wanted changes to postprocedure management of patients at the hospital level. Physicians that participated as assessors were more likely to implement changes to their practice rather that physicians that submitted cases for study. The active assessment of cases was more beneficial for physicians than getting passive feedback about improvements for individual cases.[46] This active case reflection and assessment is an important component of lifelong learning.

## COMMUNITIES OF PRACTICE AND PURSUIT OF EXPERTISE

Communities of practice exemplifies a modern form of surgical education. These focused groups of surgeons and health care providers provide forums for valuable information exchange on complex patient management, joint problem solving, and operative strategies. Commonly in an online format, communities of practice are advantageous in linking experienced global knowledge, usually in a supportive and positive manner.[47,48] If there is enough expert participation within a practice community, this can serve as a platform for achieving or maintaining expertise within a field.[41] Examples of communities of practice include the Society of Vascular Surgery Connect Open Forum and the Society of American Gastrointestinal and Endoscopic Surgeons (SAGES) Foregut Facebook group.

The development of the SAGES Masters program is an example of pursuit of expertise. Initially conceived in 2015, these courses provide a structured postgraduate education for surgeons to improve their surgical skills and knowledge.[49] The clinical topics are organized into clinical pathways: acute care surgery, bariatric, biliary, colorectal, flexible endoscopy, foregut, hernia, leadership and professional development, liver, pancreas, robotics, and solid organ.[50] Each clinical pathway has 3 distinct levels of performance: competency, proficiency, and expertise.[49] These levels are based of the Dreyfus model of adult skills acquisition: novice, advanced beginner, competency, proficiency, and expertise.[51] The curriculum of each pathway includes evaluation of anchoring procedures, core lectures, CME, review of guidelines, social medial participation, and key articles for review. As part of this program, SAGES has developed a learning management program (LMS) to track surgeons' CME credits and participation within the MASTERS course.[49]

The SAGES MASTERS program is still in development but some aspects of the course have been implemented. Many of the pathways have an associated Facebook group for participants to interact. Modeled after the successful International Hernia Collaboration Facebook group,[52] the SAGES Foregut Facebook group is a private group of vetted practicing physicians, residents, and medical students that acts as a forum for education.[53] As of November 2020, the group has more than 3000 members. The content of the group was analyzed in 2018 and it was found that more than 60% of the posts were concerning operative technique and 53% of posts had associated photographs or videos.[53] These posts generated discussions on patient management and operative skills feedback. This community of practice provides an online continuous platform for physician education that does not require physician travel. This online platform is highly accessible to all interested learners, with particular benefit to surgeons with minimal local resources for education.[53] When completed, the SAGES program will be an excellent tool in the pursuit of surgeon expertise.

## CONTINUOUS PROFESSIONAL DEVELOPMENT

The concept of CPD has been accepted as a more comprehensive tool for physician education. CPD was developed to help physicians grow in all aspects of their profession and not just the clinical portion. This educational design incorporates numerous facets of a physician's profession, including but not limited to practice management, leadership, subspecialty education, and administration.[15] At its core, CPD is individualized and learner centered. One key feature is relying on the learner to identify areas of improvement. This professional education is a lifelong endeavor, as opposed to the episodic nature of CME.[15,54] As opposed to graduate medical education, CPD is the ideal method for postresidency physicians to improve as they continue multiple years of practice.[36,55] It uses multiple different formats for learning rather than only the traditional lecture-based format.[56] Participation in professional societies and collegial interaction to solve clinical problems exemplifies some forms of CPD.[54,57] CPD is meant to create a supportive rather than punitive environment for physicians to identify areas of improvement.[15] In summary, CPD integrates the 6 core competencies, MOC, and lifelong learning and represents the future of physician learning and surgical education.

## DISCLOSURE

The authors have no financial or commercial conflicts of interest in relation to this article.

## REFERENCES

1. Sachdeva AK. Acquisition and maintenance of surgical competence. Semin Vasc Surg 2002;15(3):182–90.
2. Kohn LT, Corrigan JM, Donaldson MS, editors. To err is human: building a safer health system National Academy of Sciences. 2000. Washington, DC.
3. Choudhry NK, Fletcher RH, Soumerai SB. Systematic review: the relationship between clinical experience and quality of health care. Ann Intern Med 2005;142(4): 260–73.
4. Kauffmann RM, Landman MP, Shelton J, et al. The use of a multidisciplinary morbidity and mortality conference to incorporate ACGME general competencies. J Surg Educ 2011;68(4):303–8.
5. Chung KC, Clapham PJ, Lalonde DH. Maintenance of Certification, maintenance of public trust. Plast Reconstr Surg 2011;127(2):967–73.
6. ABMS. Guide to Medical Specialties. 2020. Available at: https://www.abms.org/media/257905/abms-guide-to-medical-specialties-2020.pdf. Accessed September 9, 2020.
7. ABMS. Frequently asked questions 2020.

8. ACGME. The Milestones Guidebook. 2020. Available at: https://www.acgme.org/Portals/0/MilestonesGuidebook.pdf. Accessed October 26, 2020.
9. Swing SR. The ACGME outcome project: retrospective and prospective. Med Teach 2007;29(7):648–54.
10. Carraccio C, Wolfsthal SD, Englander R, et al. Shifting paradigms: from Flexner to competencies. Acad Med 2002;77(5):361–7.
11. Gough I. Surgeon's education, training and continuing professional development. ANZ J Surg 2009;79(3):95.
12. Economopoulos KP, Sun R, Garvey E, et al. Coaching and mentoring modern surgeons. Bull Am Coll Surg 2014;99(8):30–5.
13. Kavic MS. Competency and the six core competencies. JSLS 2002;6(2):95–7.
14. Sachdeva AK. Surgical education to improve the quality of patient care: the role of practice-based learning and improvement. J Gastrointest Surg 2007;11(11): 1379–83.
15. Sachdeva AK. The new paradigm of continuing education in surgery. Arch Surg 2005;140(3):264–9.
16. Davis DA, Mazmanian PE, Fordis M, et al. Accuracy of physician self-assessment compared with observed measures of competence: a systematic review. JAMA 2006;296(9):1094–102.
17. Sachdeva AK, Blair PG, Lupi LK. Education and Training to Address Specific Needs During the Career Progression of Surgeons. Surg Clin North Am 2016; 96(1):115–28.
18. O'Day DM. Maintenance of certification and the outside world. Arch Ophthalmol 2004;122(5):767–9.
19. ABMS. Achieving the vision: The recommendations of the Vision Initiative Commission. 2019. Available at: https://www.abms.org/media/257884/recommendations-of-the-abms-vision-initiative-commission-action-plan.pdf. Accessed October 7, 2020.
20. Darcy M. Maintenance of certification: a primer for interventional radiologists. J Vasc Interv Radiol 2006;17(11 Pt 2):S175–81.
21. ABMS. Standards for the ABMS Program for Maintenance of Certification (MOC). 2014. Available at: https://www.abms.org/media/1109/standards-for-the-abms-program-for-moc-final.pdf. Accessed October 26, 2020.
22. Lewis FR. Maintenance of Certification: American Board of Surgery goals. Am Surg 2006;72(11):1092–6, discussion 1126-1048.
23. Davis NL, Davis DA, Johnson NM, et al. Aligning academic continuing medical education with quality improvement: a model for the 21st century. Acad Med 2013;88(10):1437–41.
24. ABS. The American Board of Surgery Continuous Certification Program. 2020. Available at: https://www.absurgery.org/xfer/cc_summary.pdf. Accessed October 7, 2020.
25. Jones AT, Kopp JP, Malangoni MA. Association Between Maintaining Certification in General Surgery and Loss-of-License Actions. JAMA 2018;320(11):1195–6.
26. Bower EA, Choi D, Becker TM, et al. Awareness of and participation in maintenance of professional certification: a prospective study. J Contin Educ Health Prof 2007;27(3):164–72.
27. Bower EA, Girard DE, Wessel K, et al. Barriers to innovation in continuing medical education. J Contin Educ Health Prof 2008;28(3):148–56.
28. Stafford RE, Dreesen EB, Charles A, et al. Free and local continuing medical education does not guarantee surgeon participation in maintenance of certification learning activities. Am Surg 2010;76(7):692–6.

29. Howard-McNatt M, Sabel M, Agnese D, et al. Maintenance of Certification and Continuing Medical Education: Are They Still Required? Ann Surg Oncol 2019; 26(12):3820–3.

30. Taylor SM. Is Maintenance of Certification Working in Surgery? Adv Surg 2018; 52(1):73–87.

31. ABS. Continuous Certification Assessment Flowchart. 2020. Available at: https://www.absurgery.org/xfer/cc_flowchart.pdf. Accessed September 9, 2020.

32. Carlson ER. Lifelong Learning: A Higher Order of Consciousness and a Construct for Faculty Development. J Oral Maxillofac Surg 2019;77(10):1967 e1961–8.

33. Brandt K. From residency to lifelong learning. J Craniofac Surg 2015;26(8): 2287–8.

34. Deci EL, Ryan RM. Handbook of self-determination research. New York: University Rochester Press; 2004.

35. van der Burgt SME, Kusurkar RA, Wilschut JA, et al. Motivational Profiles and Motivation for Lifelong Learning of Medical Specialists. J Contin Educ Health Prof 2018;38(3):171–8.

36. Sachdeva AK. Continuing professional development in the twenty-first century. J Contin Educ Health Prof 2016;36(Suppl 1):S8–13.

37. Sachdeva AK, Pellegrini CA, Johnson KA. Support for simulation-based surgical education through American College of Surgeons–accredited education institutes. World J Surg 2008;32(2):196–207.

38. ABS. Training Requirements. 2020. Available at: https://www.absurgery.org/default.jsp?certgsqe_training. Accessed September 9, 2020.

39. Sullivan S, Ruis A, Pugh C. Procedural simulations and reflective practice: meeting the need. J Laparoendosc Adv Surg Tech A 2017;27(5):455–8.

40. Cooke J, Thomas-Perez A, Rooney D, et al. Overarching themes from ACS-AEI accreditation survey best practices 2011-2019. Surgery 2020;168(5):882–7.

41. Sachdeva AK. Acquiring and maintaining lifelong expertise in surgery. Surgery 2020;167(5):787–92.

42. El-Gabri D, McDow AD, Quamme SP, et al. Surgical Coaching for Advancement of Global Surgical Skills and Capacity: A Systematic Review. J Surg Res 2020; 246:499–505.

43. Greenberg CC, Ghousseini HN, Pavuluri Quamme SR, et al. A Statewide Surgical Coaching Program Provides Opportunity for Continuous Professional Development. Ann Surg 2018;267(5):868–73.

44. Bonrath EM, Dedy NJ, Gordon LE, et al. Comprehensive Surgical Coaching Enhances Surgical Skill in the Operating Room: A Randomized Controlled Trial. Ann Surg 2015;262(2):205–12.

45. Gagnon LH, Abbasi N. Systematic review of randomized controlled trials on the role of coaching in surgery to improve learner outcomes. Am J Surg 2018;216(1): 140–6.

46. Lui CW, Boyle FM, Wysocki AP, et al. How participation in surgical mortality audit impacts surgical practice. BMC Surg 2017;17(1):42.

47. Cruess RL, Cruess SR, Steinert Y. Medicine as a Community of Practice: Implications for Medical Education. Acad Med 2018;93(2):185–91.

48. Gandamihardja TA. The role of communities of practice in surgical education. J Surg Educ 2014;71(4):645–9.

49. Jones DB, Stefanidis D, Korndorffer JR Jr, et al. SAGES University MASTERS Program: a structured curriculum for deliberate, lifelong learning. Surg Endosc 2017; 31(8):3061–71.

50. SAGES. Masters program 2020.

51. Dreyfus SE. The five-stage model of adult skill acquisition. Bull Sci Technol Soc 2004;24(3):177–81.

52. Chui P, et al. Quality Improvement Through Social Media: An Initial Look at the International Hernia Collaboration Facebook(TM) Group. 2014. Available at: https://www.sages.org/meetings/annual-meeting/abstracts-archive/quality-improvement-through-social-media-an-initial-look-at-the-international-hernia-collaboration-facebooktm-group/.

53. Jackson HT, Young MT, Rodriguez HA, et al. SAGES Foregut Surgery Masters Program: a surgeon's social media resource for collaboration, education, and professional development. Surg Endosc 2018;32(6):2800–7.

54. Drude KP, Maheu M, Hilty DM. Continuing Professional Development: Reflections on a Lifelong Learning Process. Psychiatr Clin North Am 2019;42(3):447–61.

55. Wiljer D, Tavares W, Mylopoulos M, et al. Data and Lifelong Learning Protocol: Understanding Cultural Barriers and Facilitators to Using Clinical Performance Data to Support Continuing Professional Development. J Contin Educ Health Prof 2018;38(4):293–8.

56. Stewart GD, Teoh KH, Pitts D, et al. Continuing professional development for surgeons. Surgeon 2008;6(5):288–92.

57. Gagliardi AR, Wright FC, Anderson MA, et al. The role of collegial interaction in continuing professional development. J Contin Educ Health Prof 2007;27(4):214–9.

# Moving?

## Make sure your subscription moves with you!

To notify us of your new address, find your **Clinics Account Number** (located on your mailing label above your name), and contact customer service at:

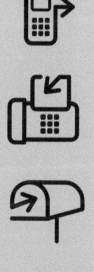

**Email: journalscustomerservice-usa@elsevier.com**

**800-654-2452** (subscribers in the U.S. & Canada)
**314-447-8871** (subscribers outside of the U.S. & Canada)

**Fax number: 314-447-8029**

**Elsevier Health Sciences Division**
**Subscription Customer Service**
**3251 Riverport Lane**
**Maryland Heights, MO 63043**

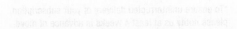